Cardiological Society of India
Yearbook of Cardiology 2023
Heart Failure

Cardiological Society of India
Yearbook of Cardiology 2023
Heart Failure

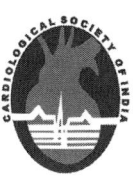

Editor-in-Chief
Roopali Khanna MD DM
Convener CSI – Heart Failure Council
Additional Professor
Department of Cardiology
Sanjay Gandhi Postgraduate Institute of Medical Sciences
Lucknow, Uttar Pradesh, India

Section Editors
Vijay Bang
PC Rath
Debabrata Roy
MK Das
PK Goel
Harikrishnan S
Tripti Deb
Satyendra Tewari
Aditya Kapoor
AK Pancholia
R Ravi Kumar
Justin Paul
Sameer Dani
Hetan C Shah

Forewords
Vijay Bang
Harikrishnan S

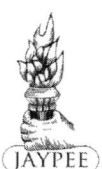

JAYPEE BROTHERS MEDICAL PUBLISHERS
The Health Sciences Publisher
New Delhi | London

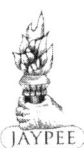 **Jaypee Brothers Medical Publishers (P) Ltd**

Headquarters
EMCA House
23/23-B, Ansari Road, Daryaganj
New Delhi 110 002, India
Landline: +91-11-23272143, +91-11-23272703
+91-11-23282021, +91-11-23245672
E-mail: jaypee@jaypeebrothers.com

Corporate Office
Jaypee Brothers Medical Publishers (P) Ltd.
4838/24, Ansari Road, Daryaganj
New Delhi 110 002, India
Phone: +91-11-43574357
Fax: +91-11-43574314
E-mail: jaypee@jaypeebrothers.com

Overseas Office
JP Medical Ltd.
83, Victoria Street, London
SW1H 0HW (UK)
Phone: +44-20 3170 8910
Fax: +44(0)20 3008 6180
E-mail: info@jpmedpub.com

Website: www.jaypeebrothers.com
Website: www.jaypeedigital.com

© 2024, Jaypee Brothers Medical Publishers and Cardiological Society of India

The views and opinions expressed in this book are solely those of the original contributor(s)/author(s) and do not necessarily represent those of editor(s) or publisher of the book.

All rights reserved. No part of this publication may be reproduced, stored or transmitted in any form or by any means, electronic, mechanical, photocopying, recording or otherwise, without the prior permission in writing of the publishers.

All brand names and product names used in this book are trade names, service marks, trademarks or registered trademarks of their respective owners. The publisher is not associated with any product or vendor mentioned in this book.

Medical knowledge and practice change constantly. This book is designed to provide accurate, authoritative information about the subject matter in question. However, readers are advised to check the most current information available on procedures included and check information from the manufacturer of each product to be administered, to verify the recommended dose, formula, method and duration of administration, adverse effects and contraindications. It is the responsibility of the practitioner to take all appropriate safety precautions. Neither the publisher nor the author(s)/editor(s) assume any liability for any injury and/or damage to persons or property arising from or related to use of material in this book.

This book is sold on the understanding that the publisher is not engaged in providing professional medical services. If such advice or services are required, the services of a competent medical professional should be sought.

Every effort has been made where necessary to contact holders of copyright to obtain permission to reproduce copyright material. If any have been inadvertently overlooked, the publisher will be pleased to make the necessary arrangements at the first opportunity.

Inquiries for bulk sales may be solicited at: jaypee@jaypeebrothers.com

CSI Yearbook of Cardiology 2023: Heart Failure / Roopali Khanna

First Edition: 2024

ISBN: 978-93-5696-613-0

Printed at Replika Press Pvt. Ltd.

Dedication

Dedicated to my teachers, my family, and the almighty.

Contributors

Editor-in-Chief

Roopali Khanna MD DM
Convener CSI – Heart Failure Council
Additional Professor
Department of Cardiology
Sanjay Gandhi Postgraduate Institute of Medical Sciences
Lucknow, Uttar Pradesh, India

Section Editors

Aditya Kapoor MD DM
Professor and Head
Department of Cardiology
Sanjay Gandhi Postgraduate Institute of Medical Sciences
Lucknow, Uttar Pradesh, India

AK Pancholia MD
Head, Medicine
Arihant Hospital
Indore, Madhya Pradesh, India

Debabrata Roy MD DM
(Cardiology) FACC FESC FSCAI FAHA
Senior Consultant
Interventional
Cardiologist and Academic
Co-ordinator
NH-RTIICS
Kolkata, West Bengal, India

Harikrishnan S DM FRCP FAMS
Professor and Head
Department of Cardiology
Sree Chitra Tirunal Institute
for Medical Sciences and
Technology
Thiruvananthapuram, Kerala,
India

Hetan C Shah MD DM
Professor
Department of Cardiology
Seth GS Medical College and
KEM Hospital
Mumbai, Maharashtra, India

Justin Paul MD DNB DM
Professor
Department of Cardiology
Madras Medical College
Chennai, Tamil Nadu, India

MK Das MD DM
Consultant Cardiologist
BM Birla and CMRI Hospitals
Kolkata, West Bengal, India

PC Rath MD DM FICC FESC FACC
FRCP (London) FRCP (Edinburgh)
Senior Consultant Cardiologist
and Head
Department of Cardiology
Apollo Hospital, Jubilee Hills
Hyderabad, Telangana
Apollo Hospital
Bhubaneswar, Odisha, India

PK Goel MD DM
Director, Interventional
Cardiology, Medanta Super
Speciality Hospital
Lucknow, Uttar Pradesh, India

R Ravi Kumar MD DM
Senior Consultant and
Associate Clinical Lead
Institute of Heart and Lung
Transplant and Mechanical
Circulatory Support
MGM Healthcare
Chennai, Tamil Nadu, India

Sameer Dani MD DM
CEO, Apollo CVHF Heart Institute
Director
Department of Cardiology
Apollo Hospital, Gandhi Nagar
Ahmedabad, Gujarat, India

Satyendra Tewari MD DM
Professor
Department of Cardiology
Sanjay Gandhi Postgraduate Institute of Medical Sciences
Lucknow, Uttar Pradesh, India

Tripti Deb MD DNB
Senior Consultant
Interventional Cardiologist
Apollo Health City
Hyderabad, Telangana, India

Vijay Bang MD DM FCSI FESC FSCAI FACC
Senior Interventional Cardiologist
Lilavati Hospital and Research Center
Honorable Professor and Head
Grant Medical College and Sir JJ Group of Hospitals (Former)
Mumbai, Maharashtra, India

Co-Editors

Akshaya Pradhan MD DM
Professor
Department of Cardiology
King George's Medical University
Lucknow, Uttar Pradesh, India

Anindya Ghosh MD DM
Associate Consultant
Department of Cardiac Electrophysiology and Pacing
Arrhythmia Heart Failure Academy
Madras Medical Mission
Chennai, Tamil Nadu, India

Arpita Katheria MD DM
Assistant Professor
Department of Cardiology
Sanjay Gandhi Postgraduate Institute of Medical Sciences
Lucknow, Uttar Pradesh, India

Atul Kaushik MD DM
Associate Professor
AIIMS
Jodhpur, Rajasthan, India

Bhuwan Chand Tewari MD DM
Professor and Head
Department of Cardiology
Dr Ram Manohar Lohia Institute of Medical Sciences
Lucknow, Uttar Pradesh, India

Daljeet Kaur Saggu MD DM
Senior Consultant
Department of Cardiology and Electrophysiology
AIG Hospitals
Hyderabad, Telangana, India

Deepchandh Raja MD DM DNB FNB
Senior Consultant Cardiologist and Clinical Lead of Cardiac Electrophysiology
Kauvery Hospital
Chennai, Tamil Nadu, India

Harshit Khare MD DM
Assistant Professor
Department of Cardiology
Sanjay Gandhi Postgraduate Institute of Medical Sciences
Lucknow, Uttar Pradesh, India

Kavita Tyagi MD DNB
Consultant
Department of Cardiology
Sir Ganga Ram Hospital
New Delhi, India

Linda Koshy PhD
Scientist B
Sree Chitra Tirunal Institute for Medical Sciences and Technology
Thiruvananthapuram, Kerala, India

Mahpaekar Mashhadi MD DM
Consultant Interventional Cardiologist
Apollo CVHF Heart Institute
Ahmedabad, Gujarat, India

Manik Chopra MD DM
Clinical Lead, Structural Heart Disease Interventions (TAVR)
Narayana Multispeciality Hospitals
Ahmedabad, Gujarat, India

Manojit Lodha MD DM
Associate Professor
RKM Seva Pratishthan, VIMS
Kolkata, West Bengal, India

Mona Bhatia MD DM
Principal Director and Head
Department of Radiology and Imaging
Fortis Escorts Heart Institute and Research Centre
New Delhi, India

Muthiah Subramaniam MD DM
Consultant
Department of Cardiology
AIG Hospital
Hyderabad, Telangana, India

Poonam Tripathi PhD
Research Associate
Department of Cardiology
Sanjay Gandhi Postgraduate Institute of Medical Sciences
Lucknow, Uttar Pradesh, India

Prayaag Kinni MD DNB
Consultant Cardiologist
Sri Sathya Sai Institute of Higher Medical Sciences
Bengaluru, Karnataka, India

Shantanu Sengupta MD DNB FCCP
Consultant
Sengupta Hospital and Research Institute
Nagpur, Maharashtra, India

Sharad Chandra MD DM
Professor
Department of Cardiology
King George's Medical University
Lucknow, Uttar Pradesh, India

Sudeep Kumar MD DM
Professor
Department of Cardiology
Sanjay Gandhi Postgraduate Institute of Medical Sciences
Lucknow, Uttar Pradesh, India

Suman Jatain MD DM
Associate Consultant
Department of Cardiology
Max Healthcare
New Delhi, India

Sumit Rakshit
Postdoctoral Fellow
NH-RTIICS
Kolkata, West Bengal, India

Surendra Deora MD DM
Additional Professor
Department of Cardiology
AIIMS
Jodhpur, Rajasthan, India

Foreword

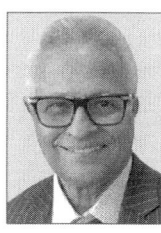

Vijay Bang MD DM FCSI FESC FSCAI FACC
Senior Interventional Cardiologist
Lilavati Hospital and Research Center, Mumbai, Maharashtra, India
President, CSI 2023 (Platinum Jubilee)
President-Elect and Chairman, Scientific Committee
CSI Annual Conference 2022 at Chennai
Honorary Professor and Head, Grant Government Medical College and
Sir JJ Group of Hospitals, Mumbai (Former)
- Founding President, Cardiovascular Academic Research Foundation
- Founding Course Director, India Act Conference
- Founding Director and Moderator, International Cardiology CME
- Founding Course Director, National Cardiology PG Course

I am happy to write foreword for "*CSI Yearbook of Heart Failure 2023*" which being published by a group of experts in the field of heart failure. The authors have picked up landmark articles with good clinical relevance from high-impact medical journals with special emphasis on the articles from the Indian subcontinent. This comprehensive collection of articles will enable our cardiology fellows and practicing physicians to get an overview of the new developments in the field of heart failure. The abstracts of the article tell us the science and evidence on the topic. The commentaries give you an expert's opinion on interpreting these trials published in 2022–2023.

Heart failure remains a global health challenge, affecting millions of individuals and burdening healthcare systems around the world. In today's era of advancement and digital technology, a physician needs to be aware of the latest developments in various fields. This helps in taking better care of the patient and improving the outcomes. In this collection of articles, authors delve into the most recent advancements in our understanding of heart failure, the innovative approaches to diagnosis, the evolving landscape of heart failure management, the impact of digital health technologies, and the exploration of innovative treatments. The insights into the molecular and genetic underpinnings of heart failure, and strategies to address heart failure disparities in different populations are also discussed. Precision medicine and patient-centered care in heart failure management are the paths of the future and will be a reality in the coming years.

The quest for knowledge is a perpetual one, and this book is a remarkable testament of our collective commitment to improving the care and outcomes of heart failure patients. As we read these articles and commentaries, we are presented with a tapestry of discoveries in diagnosis and treatment.

I hope this exercise will continue in the coming years and we wish good luck to the editors for this.

Foreword

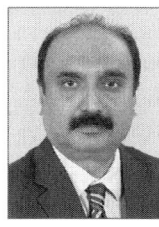

Harikrishnan S DM FRCP FAMS
Editor-in-Chief: Heart Failure Journal of India
PI–ICMR National Center for Research and Excellence in Heart Failure
Professor and Head, Department of Cardiology
Sree Chitra Tirunal Institute for Medical Sciences and Technology
Thiruvananthapuram, Kerala, India

The arena of heart failure (HF) has witnessed very remarkable developments in the last few years with more and more therapies emerging, which have shown to improve the survival and quality of life among patients affected with the disease. Indian cardiology community has also made significant contributions by generating data through registries and also being part of many major clinical trials. The data from these registries have shown that our patients are younger and their short-term and long-term outcomes are worse compared to other regions of the world. Accessibility, availability, and affordability issues affect the quality of care received by patients with HF. System and physician inertia is one important issue which is affecting HF care in India.

Initiatives like publication of a 'Yearbook' highlighting the developments in the different facets of HF become important in this background. As the clinical workload is high, many practicing physicians find it difficult to keep abreast with the latest developments in HF. As we have witnessed over the last few years, there has been a tremendous change with many new drugs being added to the therapeutic armamentarium of HF. So, initiatives like this will help them to get acquainted with the emerging data on evaluation and management of HF.

Dr Roopali Khanna must be congratulated for leading this initiative of Cardiological Society of India (CSI). This book has 12 Sections covering different aspects of HF, including arrhythmias, genetics, drug therapy, cardiomyopathy, HF in women, digital technology, imaging, interventions, and advanced treatment in HF, including cardiac transplantation. The editor and the authors have done a wonderful job in collecting the most outstanding literature in the previous year and presenting in a simple but elegant format.

I am sure it will be a very good read for the busy clinician, resident trainees, and fellows in cardiology alike. I am certain that the reader will get the information to refine his management plan for patients with HF, which is becoming more and more complex. I am sure the readers will surely await the coming year's yearbook and I wish this publication all the very best.

Preface

Exploring the Complex Landscape of Heart Failure

Heart failure, a multifaceted cardiovascular condition, continues to be a prominent concern in the realm of modern medicine. Recent advancements in research and clinical practice have shed new light on the intricacies of heart failure, unveiling innovative approaches for diagnosis, treatment, and prevention. This "CSI Yearbook of Heart Failure 2023" is a collection of articles that delve into the latest discoveries and developments in the field, aiming to provide readers with a comprehensive overview of heart failure research and care.

We have tried to include impactful scientific data published in 2022–2023. There are 12 sections with experts in the respective fields as editors. Each section has approximately 6 articles from high-impact journals. The diverse range of topics explored by experts in the area, from cutting-edge diagnostic techniques and novel therapeutic interventions to the growing significance of digital technology in managing heart failure. The abstract provides the original data, and its interpretation is given by the experts in the commentaries. Due to copyright issues, the abstracts have been rephrased, retaining the central message of the trial. A title is given to each commentary, which provides the central message of the trial. The commentary discusses the article and relevant issues emphasising the current evidence-based thinking on the subject. We hope these articles serve as a valuable resource for cardiology fellows and practicing physicians seeking to enhance their understanding of heart failure and its management. A special section on recent heart failure guidelines provides 10 key messages from the experts.

I have no words to express my gratitude to the editors and the sub-editors who put in so much effort for this endeavour. A special thanks to Dr Harshit Khare and Dr Arpita Katheria, who spent many hours searching and compiling the articles. Dr Poonam Tripathi and Mr Tapish Srivastava, my office team, coordinated all the activities, and without them, this book would not have been possible. Grateful to the Jaypee brothers for providing the required logistics to make this book possible. Pallavi A Mehrotra, Development Editor, Jaypee Brothers Medical Publishers, is a competent, patient and delightful to work with.

We hope that the information and insights shared in these articles will improve our knowledge in the management of heart failure patients and inspire further research and innovative practices.

Roopali Khanna

Acknowledgments

I want to express my heartfelt thanks and appreciation to all the section editors and associate editors who played a significant role in the creation of this book. Their expertise and guidance was indispensable. I am grateful to the Cardiological Society of India (CSI), President Dr Vijay Bang, and Honorary General Secretary Dr Debabrata Roy for their unwavering support, encouragement, and valuable insights throughout the writing process.

I also extend my appreciation to Shri Jitendar P Vij (Group Chairman), Mr Ankit Vij (Managing Director), Mr MS Mani (Group President), Ms Chetna Malhotra (Senior Director—Professional Publishing, Marketing, and Business Development), Ms Pooja Bhandari [Director—Production (Books and Journals)], Pallavi A Mehrotra (Development Editor), and the publishing team at Jaypee Brothers Medical Publishers (P) Ltd for their professionalism and dedication in bringing this book to life. Special thanks to my family, friends, and loved ones for their patience and for bearing with me during the long hours I spent working on this project. Lastly, I want to thank the readers interested in this field of work. This book would not have been possible without the collective efforts and support of these wonderful individuals and organization. Thank you all for making this possible.

Roopali Khanna

Contents

Section 1: Guidelines/Consensus Document
Section Editors: Debabrata Roy, PC Rath, Vijay Bang
Co-Editor: Sumit Rakshit

1. Supervised Exercise Training for Chronic Heart Failure with Preserved Ejection Fraction: A Scientific Statement from the American Heart Association and American College of Cardiology — 1
2. 2022 AHA/ACC/HFSA Guideline for the Management of Heart Failure — 3
3. 2023 ACC Expert Consensus Decision Pathway on Management of Heart Failure With Preserved Ejection Fraction: A Report of the American College of Cardiology Solution Set Oversight Committee — 4

Section 2: Epidemiology in Heart Failure
Section Editor: Satyendra Tewari
Co-Editor: Harshit Khare

1. Cigarette Smoking, Cessation, and Risk of Heart Failure with Preserved and Reduced Ejection Fraction — 6
2. Natural History and Prognostic Significance of Iron Deficiency and Anemia in Ambulatory Patients with Chronic Heart Failure — 8
3. Impact of Moderate Aortic Stenosis in Patients with Heart Failure with Reduced Ejection Fraction — 10
4. Cardiogenic Shock from Heart Failure versus Acute Myocardial Infarction: Clinical Characteristics, Hospital Course, and 1-year Outcomes — 12

Section 3: Imaging in Heart Failure
Section Editor: MK Das
Co-Editors: Shantanu Sengupta, Mona Bhatia

1. Quantified Mitral Regurgitation and Left Atrial Function in Heart Failure with Reduced Ejection Fraction: Interplay and Outcome Implications — 16
2. Clinical Implications of Left Atrial Changes after Optimization of Medical Therapy in Patients with Heart Failure — 19

3.	Strain Echocardiography in Predicting LV Dysfunction in RV Apical Pacing	20
4.	Left Ventricular Global Longitudinal Strain Imaging in Identifying Subclinical Myocardial Dysfunction Among COVID-19 Survivors	21
5.	Prognostic Value of Global Longitudinal Strain in Patients with Heart Failure with Improved Ejection Fraction	22
6.	Right Ventricular Dysfunction in Patients with New-onset Heart Failure: Longitudinal Follow-up during Guideline-directed Medical Therapy	24
7.	Correlation of Serum ST2 Levels with Severity of Diastolic Dysfunction on Echocardiography and Findings on Cardiac MRI in Patients with Heart Failure with Preserved Ejection Fraction	25
8.	Artificial Intelligence for Contrast-free MRI: Scar Assessment in Myocardial Infarction using Deep Learning-based Virtual Native Enhancement	27
9.	Validating an Idiopathic Dilated Cardiomyopathy Diagnosis using Cardiovascular Magnetic Resonance: The Dilated Cardiomyopathy Precision Medicine Study	30
10.	Cardiac Magnetic Resonance Identifies Raised Left Ventricular Filling Pressure: Prognostic Implications	32

Section 4: Genetics in Heart Failure
Section Editor: Harikrishnan S
Co-Editors: Sudeep Kumar, Linda Koshy, Poonam Tripathi

1.	Risk Prognostication with Genotype versus Phenotype in Genetic Cardiomyopathies	35
2.	Genotyping Indian Patients with Primary Cardiomyopathies-analysis of Database	37
3.	Clinical Risk Score to Predict Pathogenic Genotypes in Patients with Dilated Cardiomyopathy	39
4.	Genetic Architecture of Acute Myocarditis and the Overlap with Inherited Cardiomyopathy	40
5.	The Response to Cardiac Resynchronization Therapy in LMNA Cardiomyopathy	43

Section 5: Drug Therapy in Heart Failure
Section Editor: AK Pancholia
Co-Editor: Akshaya Pradhan

1.	Dapagliflozin in Heart Failure with Mildly Reduced or Preserved Ejection Fraction: DELIVER Trial	46
2.	Combining Loop with Thiazide Diuretics for Decompensated Heart Failure: The CLOROTIC Trial	48
3.	Acetazolamide in Decompensated Heart Failure with Volume Overload: The ADVOR Trial	50
4.	Effects of Empagliflozin on Symptoms, Physical Limitations, and Quality of Life in Patients Hospitalized for Acute Heart Failure: Results from the EMPULSE Trial	52

5. Torsemide Comparison with Furosemide for Management of Heart Failure: TRANSFORM-HF Trial — 55
6. Virtual Care Team-guided Strategy Optimizes GDMT for Hospitalized HF Patients: The IMPLEMENT-HF Trial — 57
7. Effect of Sacubitril/Valsartan versus Valsartan on Left Atrial Volume in Patients with Pre-heart Failure with Preserved Ejection Fraction: The PARABLE Randomized Clinical Trial — 59
8. Effect of Omecamtiv Mecarbil on Exercise Capacity in Chronic Heart Failure with Reduced Ejection Fraction: The METEORIC-HF Randomized Clinical Trial — 61
9. Study of Dietary Sodium Intervention Under 100 mmol in Heart Failure (SODIUM-HF): An International, Open-label, Randomized, Controlled Trial — 63
10. Electronic Alerts to Improve Heart Failure Therapy in Outpatient Practice: A Cluster Randomized Trial — 66
11. Safety, Tolerability, and Efficacy of Up-titration of Guideline-directed Medical Therapies for Acute Heart Failure (STRONG-HF): A Multinational, Open-label, Randomized Trial — 68
12. Patiromer for the Management of Hyperkalemia in Heart Failure with Reduced Ejection Fraction: The DIAMOND Trial — 70
13. Tolvaptan Add-on Therapy and Its Effects on Efficacy Parameters and Outcomes in Patients Hospitalized with Heart Failure — 72
14. β3 Adrenergic Agonist Treatment in Chronic Pulmonary Hypertension Associated with Heart Failure (SPHERE-HF): A Double Blind, Placebo-controlled, Randomized Clinical Trial — 74
15. Effects of Sildenafil on Symptoms and Exercise Capacity for Heart Failure with Reduced Ejection Fraction and Pulmonary Hypertension (The SilHF Study): A Randomized Placebo Controlled Multicentre Trial — 76
16. Empagliflozin in Acute Myocardial Infarction: The EMMY Trial — 79

Section 6: Cardiomyopathy
Section Editor: Sameer Dani
Co-Editors: Mahpaekar Mashhadi, Bhuwan Chand Tewari

1. Dose-blinded Myosin Inhibition in Patients with Obstructive Hypertrophic Cardiomyopathy Referred for Septal Reduction Therapy: Outcomes through 32 Weeks — 82
2. Survival Following Alcohol Septal Ablation or Septal Myectomy for Patients with Obstructive Hypertrophic Cardiomyopathy — 84
3. Systemic Embolism, a Dreaded Complication in Amyloid Transthyretin Cardiomyopathy — 86
4. Structural and Functional Brain Changes in Acute Takotsubo Syndrome — 87
5. The Prevalence and Association of Exercise Test Abnormalities with Sudden Cardiac Death and Transplant-free Survival in Childhood Hypertrophic Cardiomyopathy — 89

Section 7: Arrhythmia and Heart Failure
Section Editor: Aditya Kapoor
Co-Editors: Deepchandh Raja, Daljeet Kaur Saggu, Muthiah Subramaniam, Anindya Ghosh

1. Incidence of Sudden Cardiac Death and Life-threatening Arrhythmias in Clinically Manifest Cardiac Sarcoidosis with and without Current Indications for an Implantable Cardioverter Defibrillator — 92
2. Randomized Trial of Left Bundle Branch versus Biventricular Pacing for Cardiac Resynchronization Therapy — 94
3. Predictors for Early Mortality in Patients with Implantable Cardiac Defibrillator for Heart Failure with Reduced Ejection Fraction — 96
4. Predictors of Primary Prevention Implantable Cardioverter-defibrillator Use in Heart Failure with Reduced Ejection Fraction: Impact of the Predicted Risk of Sudden Cardiac Death and All-cause Mortality — 98
5. Cardioverter-defibrillator Reduces Mortality Risk in Eligible Ischemic and Nonischemic Cardiomyopathy Patients: Sub-analysis of the Multicenter Improve SCA Study — 100
6. Rivaroxaban in Rheumatic Heart Disease-associated Atrial Fibrillation — 101
7. Randomized Ablation-based Rhythm-control versus Rate-control Trial in Patients with Heart Failure and Atrial Fibrillation: Results from the RAFT-AF trial — 104

Section 8: Heart Failure in Women
Section Editor: Justin Paul
Co-Editor: Arpita Katheria

1. Infertility and Risk of Heart Failure in the Women's Health Initiative — 107
2. Distinct Pathophysiological Pathways in Women and Men with Heart Failure — 109
3. Heart Failure Subtypes and Cardiomyopathies in Women — 111
4. Pregnancy Outcomes in Women with Heart Disease: The Madras Medical College Pregnancy and Cardiac (M-PAC) Registry from India — 113
5. Focused Cardiac Ultrasound to Guide the Diagnosis of Heart Failure in Pregnant Women in India — 115

Section 9: Advance Therapy in the Management of Heart Failure
Section Editor: R Ravi Kumar
Co-Editors: Surendra Deora, Kavita Tyagi

1. Five-year Outcomes in Patients with Fully Magnetically Levitated versus Axial-flow Left Ventricular Assist Devices in the MOMENTUM 3 Randomized Trial — 118
2. Right Heart Failure Following Left Ventricular Device Implantation: Natural History, Risk Factors, and Outcomes: An Analysis of the STS INTERMACS Database — 120

3. Renal Sympathetic Denervation in Patients with Heart Failure with Preserved
   Ejection Fraction — 121
4. Renal Compression in Heart Failure: The Renal Tamponade Hypothesis — 124
5. Riociguat in Pulmonary Hypertension and Heart Failure with Preserved
   Ejection Fraction: The HemoDYNAMIC Trial — 125
6. Randomized Trial of Targeted Transendocardial Mesenchymal Precursor
   Cell Therapy in Patients with Heart Failure — 127
7. Cardiac Contractility Modulation Therapy Improves Health Status in Patients with
   Heart Failure with Preserved Ejection Fraction: A Pilot Study (CCM-HFpEF) — 129
8. Baroreflex Activation Therapy with the Barostim™ Device in Patients with
   Heart Failure with Reduced Ejection Fraction: A Patient Level Meta-analysis of
   Randomized Controlled Trials — 131

Section 10: Interventions in Heart Failure
Section Editor: PK Goel
Co-Editors: Manik Chopra, Atul Kaushik

1. Hospitalizations and Mortality in Patients with Secondary Mitral Regurgitation and
   Heart Failure: The COAPT Trial — 134
2. Percutaneous Revascularization for Ischemic Left Ventricular Dysfunction — 136
3. Intermittent Occlusion of the Superior Vena Cava to Improve
   Hemodynamics in Patients with Acutely Decompensated Heart Failure:
   The VENUS-HF Early Feasibility Study — 138
4. Durability of Benefit after Transcatheter Tricuspid Valve Intervention:
   Insights from Actigraphy — 140
5. Left Atrial Volume Index and Outcome after Transcatheter Edge-to-edge Valve
   Repair for Secondary Mitral Regurgitation — 142
6. Transcatheter Repair for Patients with Tricuspid Regurgitation — 144
7. Transcatheter Mitral Valve Replacement or Repair for Secondary Mitral Regurgitation:
   A Propensity Score-matched Analysis — 146

Section 11: Digital Technology in Heart Failure
Section Editor: Hetan C Shah
Co-Editors: Prayaag Kinni, Manojit Lodha

1. Artificial Intelligence in Cardiovascular Medicine: Current Insights and Future Prospects — 148
2. Electronic Alerts to Improve Heart Failure Therapy in Outpatient Practice a Cluster
   Randomized Trial — 149
3. Machine Learning-based Prediction of Myocardial Recovery in Patients with
   Left Ventricular Assist Device Support — 152

4. Device-based Remote Monitoring Strategies for Congestion-guided
   Management of Patients with Heart Failure: A Systematic Review and Meta-analysis ... 153
5. Applications of Machine Learning in Cardiology ... 154
6. Effects of Remote Hemodynamic-guided Heart Failure Management in
   Patients with Different Subtypes of Pulmonary Hypertension: Insights from the
   MEMS-HF Study ... 155
7. Longer-term Effects of Remote Patient Management Following Hospital
   Discharge after Acute Systolic Heart Failure: The Randomized E-INH Trial ... 157

Section 12: Miscellaneous
Section Editor: Tripti Deb
Co-Editors: Sharad Chandra, Suman Jatain

1. Nutrition Assessment and Dietary Interventions in Heart Failure JACC
   Review Topic of the Week ... 160
2. Spirituality in Patients with Heart Failure ... 162
3. Intravenous Ferric Derisomaltose in Patients with Heart Failure and Iron
   Deficiency in the UK (IRONMAN): An Investigator-initiated, Prospective,
   Randomized, Open-label, Blinded-endpoint Trial ... 164
4. Impact of Ischemic Etiology on the Efficacy of Intravenous Ferric
   Carboxymaltose in Patients with Iron Deficiency and Acute Heart Failure:
   Insights from the AFFIRM-AHF Trial ... 167
5. Outcome of Heart Failure Management in a Multidisciplinary Clinic:
   A Randomized Controlled Trial ... 169
6. Albuminuria as a Marker of Systemic Congestion in Patients with Heart Failure ... 171

Index ... ***175***

SECTION 1

Guidelines/Consensus Document

Section Editors: **Vijay Bang, PC Rath, Debabrata Roy**

Co-Editor: **Sumit Rakshit**

ARTICLE 1

Supervised Exercise Training for Chronic Heart Failure with Preserved Ejection Fraction: A Scientific Statement from the American Heart Association and American College of Cardiology

Sachdev V, Sharma K, Keteyian SJ, Alcain CF, Desvigne-Nickens P, Fleg JL, et al.; American Heart Association Heart Failure and Transplantation Committee of the Council on Clinical Cardiology; Council on Arteriosclerosis, Thrombosis and Vascular Biology; and American College of Cardiology (2023). Supervised Exercise Training for Chronic Heart Failure With Preserved Ejection Fraction: A Scientific Statement From the American Heart Association and American College of Cardiology.
Circulation. 2023;147(16):e699–e715.

The 10 key messages from this scientific statement are:

1. Heart failure with preserved ejection fraction (HFpEF) is a prevalent and worsening form of HF, causing severe exertional dyspnea, fatigue, poor quality of life, frequent hospitalizations with high mortality rates and has severely reduced aerobic exercise capacity as well, due to several pathophysiological mechanisms involving skeletal muscle, cardiac, pulmonary, and vascular systems. These with other contributing factors such as sedentary behavior, atrial fibrillation and obesity leads to increased plasma volume, pericardial restraint, and cardiac remodeling. Intra-abdominal adiposity, in particular, is crucial in its pathogenesis and is associated with widespread systemic inflammation, capillary rarefaction, mitochondrial dysfunction, and decreased bioavailability of nitric oxide.

2. While pharmacological trials for HFpEF showed neutral outcomes, exercise-based trials consistently demonstrated significant and clinically meaningful improvements in symptoms, exercise capacity, and quality of life. The positive effects of exercise can be attributed to its pleiotropic impacts on various abnormalities in peripheral vascular, skeletal muscle, and cardiovascular systems.

3. Impairments in the physiological reserve capacity of numerous organ systems

characterize exercise intolerance in HFpEF; however, the relative cardiac and extracardiac deficiencies differ between people.[1] Exercise training in HFpEF reported improvements in diastolic function measures and peripheral adaptations in skeletal muscles. The changes in peripheral adaptations, such as increased mitochondrial density and function, myoglobin content, capillary density, blood flow redistribution, diffusion capacity and oxygen extraction by muscles may contribute to the observed improvements in peak VO_2.

4. *Exercise training may be*:
   - Self-directed exercise training (Performed without supervision or formal exercise prescription): Current guidelines recommend ≥150 min/week of moderate-intensity physical activity and ≥2 days/week of muscle-strengthening activities. However, there are no specific data on the safety and efficacy of self-directed exercise in patients with HFpEF.
   - *Structured exercise training (SET)*: It is typically conducted in a clinical setting with monitoring and includes at least three sessions per week of aerobic-type exercises like walking or stationary cycling. Muscle strengthening may also be included, and 36 visits are generally prescribed within a 12-week period.

5. Studies on exercise training in patients with HFpEF excluded patients with common comorbidities such as atrial fibrillation, chronic obstructive pulmonary disease, and coronary artery disease as well as certain demographic groups, such as older adults, women, individuals with lower socioeconomic status, and underrepresented racial and ethnic groups. This exclusion could limit the generalizability of the results of exercise training to a broader HFpEF population.

6. Various approaches for training, including walking, stationary cycle ergometry, high-intensity interval training (HIIT), strength training, and dancing were utilized. The primary outcome measures for most trials were exercise capacity parameters such as peak VO_2, exercise test time, and 6-minute walk distance (6MWD). These outcome measures are important for improving physical function and quality of life in patients with HFpEF, which is a significant improvement given their chronic symptoms and reduced quality of life.

7. The meta-analysis of the included randomized controlled trials (RCTs) showed that aerobic exercise training significantly improved peak VO_2, total exercise test time, and 6MWD in patients with HFpEF. The improvements observed in peak VO_2 ranged from 12 to 14%, which is considered clinically meaningful. However, the duration of most trials was relatively short (3-6 months), and long-term maintenance of the benefits remains a challenge.

8. The safety of exercise training in HFpEF has been consistently demonstrated with no exercise-related major adverse events reported in the trials. Adherence to the exercise programs varied but was generally acceptable with completion rates ranging from 76 to 90%. However, long-term adherence remains a challenge, and future studies should address strategies to improve adherence.

9. Studies combining aerobic exercise training with caloric restriction in obese *HFpEF* patients showed independent

and additive benefits. Both interventions resulted in weight loss and improvements in peak VO$_2$ and quality-of-life measures.

10. A few trials of home-based exercise training in HFpEF patients demonstrated improved exercise capacity and quality of life. Hybrid models that combine facility-based and home-based exercise

ARTICLE 2

2022 AHA/ACC/HFSA Guideline for the Management of Heart Failure

ACC/AHA Joint Committee Members. 2022 AHA/ACC/HFSA Guideline for the Management of Heart Failure. *J Card Fail.* 2022;28(5):e1-e167.

■ CONGESTIVE HEART FAILURE GUIDELINE-DIRECTED MEDICAL THERAPY: TEN COMMANDMENTS

1. Guideline-directed medical therapy (GDMT) for heart failure with reduced ejection fraction (HFrEF) now includes four medication classes which include sodium-glucose cotransporter-2 inhibitors (SGLT-2Is).
2. SGLT-2Is have a 2a recommendation in heart failure with mildly reduced ejection fraction (HFmrEF). Weaker recommendations (2b) are made for angiotensin-receptor-neprilysin inhibitor (ARNI), angiotensin-converting enzyme inhibitor (ACEI), angiotensin receptor blocker (ARB), mineralocorticoid receptor antagonist (MRA) and β-blockers in this population.
3. New recommendations for HFpEF are made for SGLT-2Is (2a), MRAs (2b), and ARNI (2b). Several prior recommendations have been renewed including treatment of hypertension (1), treatment of atrial fibrillation (2a), use of ARBs (2b) avoidance of routine use of nitrates or phosphodiesterase-5 inhibitors (3-no benefit).
4. Improved left ventricular ejection fraction (LVEF) is used to refer to those patients with a previous HFrEF who now have a LVEF > 40%. These patients should continue their HFrEF treatment.
5. Value statements were created for select recommendations where high-quality cost effectiveness studies of the intervention have been published.
6. Amyloid heart disease has new recommendations for treatment including screening for serum and urine monoclonal light chains, bone scintigraphy, genetic sequencing, tetramer stabilizer therapy, and anticoagulation.
7. Evidence supporting increased filling pressures is important for the diagnosis of HF if the LVEF > 40%. Evidence for increased filling pressures can be obtained from noninvasive (e.g., natriuretic peptide and diastolic function on imaging) or invasive testing (e.g., hemodynamic measurements).

8. Patients with advanced HF who wish to prolong survival should be referred to a team specializing in HF. HF specialty team reviews HF management, assesses suitability for advanced HF therapies, and uses palliative care including palliative ionotropes where consistent with the patient's goals of care.
9. Primary prevention is important for those at risk for HF (Stage A) or pre-HF (Stage B). Stages of HF were reviewed to emphasize the new terminologies of "at risk" for HF for Stage A and Pre-HF for Stage B.
10. Recommendations are provided for select patients with HF and iron deficiency, anemia, hypertension, sleep disorders, type 2 diabetes mellitus, atrial fibrillation, coronary artery disease, and malignancy.

ARTICLE 3

2023 ACC Expert Consensus Decision Pathway on Management of Heart Failure With Preserved Ejection Fraction: A Report of the American College of Cardiology Solution Set Oversight Committee

Kittleson MM, Panjrath GS, Amancherla K, et al. 2023 ACC Expert Consensus Decision Pathway on Management of Heart Failure With Preserved Ejection Fraction: A Report of the American College of Cardiology Solution Set Oversight Committee.
J Am Coll Cardiol. 2023;81(18):1835-78.

The 10 key messages of 2023 ACC expert consensus decision pathway on management of heart failure with preserved ejection fraction (HFpEF):
1. A multidisciplinary approach is essential in diagnosing and managing HFpEF patients including primary physicians, cardiology specialists, HF specialists, and multidisciplinary specialists.
2. The H_2FPEF and HFpEF scores have some caveats and need to be clinically correlated before excluding or diagnosing HFpEF.
3. Compared to men, women have more attributable risk factors with unique sex-specific risk factors (preeclampsia and central obesity) which lead to more symptoms of dyspnea.
4. Detailed history and clinical examination and, if needed, diagnostic tests to be done to rule out HFpEF mimics (infiltrative disorders, high output states, hypertrophic cardiomyopathy, etc.)
5. Management of HFpEF needs to be done in three categories (a) risk stratification and management of comorbidities, (b) nonpharmacological management in the form of weight control and exercise, and (c) pharmacological treatment.
6. Sodium-glucose cotransporter-2 inhibitor (SGLT-2I) has shown a significant reduction in HF hospitalization and

mortality and should be given in patients of HFpEF. (Class IIa)
7. Mineralocorticoid receptor antagonists and angiotensin receptor-neprilysin inhibitor (ARNI) may be added in women with HFpEF and in men with left ventricular ejection fraction (LVEF) < 55–60%. (Class IIb)
8. Loop diuretics to be added in patients with volume overload and NYHA II–IV.
9. Pulmonary artery pressure sensor monitoring may be implanted in selected subsets of patients (recurrent hospitalization for HF despite optimal guideline-directed medical therapy (GDMT), significant liability in volume status despite close ambulatory monitoring, cardiorenal syndrome, differentiation of HF from other causes of dyspnea is difficult.
10. A team-based approach is helpful in managing cases of HFpEF by identifying the risk factors in these cases and referring them to a cardiologist and heart failure specialist accordingly.

REFERENCES

1. Nayor M, Houstis NE, Namasivayam M, Rouvina J, Hardin C, Shah RV, et al. Impaired Exercise Tolerance in Heart Failure With Preserved Ejection Fraction: Quantification of Multiorgan System Reserve Capacity. JACC Heart Fail. 2020;8(8): 605-17.

SECTION 2

Epidemiology in Heart Failure

Section Editor: Satyendra Tewari

Co-Editor: Harshit Khare

ARTICLE 1

Cigarette Smoking, Cessation, and Risk of Heart Failure With Preserved and Reduced Ejection Fraction

Ding N, Shah AM, Blaha MJ, Chang PP, Rosamond WD, Matsushita K. Cigarette Smoking, Cessation, and Risk of Heart Failure With Preserved and Reduced Ejection Fraction.
J Am Coll Cardiol. 2022;79(23):2298-305.

Abstract

Background: A well-recognized risk factor for heart failure (HF) is "smoking". However, prospective association of cigarette smoking and smoking cessation with heart failure with preserved ejection fraction (HFpEF) and heart failure with reduced ejection fraction (HFrEF) as distinct phenotypes was evaluated by few studies.

Objectives: Present study aimed to evaluate the association of cigarette smoking and smoking cessation with the incidence of HFpEF and HFrEF.

Methods: At baseline in 2005 (age range 61–81 years) in 9,345 ARIC (Atherosclerosis Risk in Communities) study White and Black participants without history of HF were included, using multivariable Cox models they computed the associations of several established cigarette smoking parameters (smoking status, pack-years, intensity, duration, and years since cessation) with physician-adjudicated incident acute decompensated HF.

Results: There were 1,215 incident HF cases over an average follow-up of 13 years. With adjusted HRs ~2, compared with never smokers, current cigarette smoking was similarly associated with HFpEF and HFrEF. For pack-years of smoking and HF, there was observed a dose response relationship. With a lower risk of HF, a more extended period of smoking cessation was associated, but for HFpEF and HFrEF significantly elevated risk persisted up to a few decades.

Conclusion: Significant and similar associations with HFpEF and HFrEF are shown by all cigarette smoking parameters HF smoking cessation significantly reduced the risk, but for a few decades excess HF risk persisted. Smoking is an important modifiable risk factor for HF and importances of smoking prevention were highlighted and cessations for the prevention of HF, including HFpEF are well explained by resulted evidence from current study.

ARTICLE COMMENTARY

Objective: The study investigated the association of cigarette smoking with incidence of acutely decompensated heart failure (HF), reclassified either as heart failure with preserved ejection fraction (HFpEF) or with reduced ejection fraction (HFrEF) and impact of smoking cessation, if any.

The database is based on ARIC (Atherosclerosis Risk in Communities) study, that was updated in 2005 to include risk factors for HF. The present study is derived from original ARIC study population, enrolling 9,345 participants, who were followed from January 2005 to December 2019, for incidence of acute decompensated heart failure (ADHF) and cigarette smoking related parameters.

This study was restricted to investigate cigarette smoking as exposure. Smoking duration was quantified as pack-years of smoking, and separated into categories <10, 10 to <25, 25 to <40, >40 years. Similarly, years past smoking cessation was categorized as <10, 10 to <20, 20 to <30, >30 years. Covariates like age, sex, drinking habits, body mass index, blood pressure, total cholesterol, glomerular filtration rate, antihypertensives, diabetes status, cholesterol lowering medications, history of coronary heart disease (CHD) were also determined. Outcomes included acutely decompensated HF, stable chronic HF, or unclassifiable HF. Further, HF was reclassified as HFrEF (LVEF < 50%) or HFpEF (LVEF > 50%).

During median follow-up of 13 years, the multivariate-adjusted incidence rate of ADHF per 1,000 person-years was 9.7 among never smokers, 13.5 among former smokers and 20.1 among current smokers, with hazard ratio of 1.36 in former smokers and 2.36 in current smokers compared to never smokers. The results were similar for both HFrEF and HFpEF categories. Smoking in terms of pack-years showed dose-graded relationship. Those with ≥25 pack-years of smoking, had twofold increased risk for HF compared with never smokers. Pack-years between 10 and 25 years was associated with mean increase in HF and those with pack-years <10 years, were not at increased risk of HF. Similarly, long-term (>30 years) of smoking cessation was associated with 50% lower risk for HF, for both HF phenotypes, compared to current smokers. However, the elevated risk for both HFpEF and HFrEF persisted for those with 20 to <30 years of smoking cessation.

In this study, at the baseline, smokers already had higher burden of CHD. This means that they were bound to have more incidence of ADHF anyway, provided they survived the adverse cardiovascular events. This explains the mechanism of HFrEF with smoking to some extent. A more detailed subgroup analysis for the etiology of HF would have provided more insights into this. But, if we put aside this fact, the study provides enough substantial proof to consolidate the fact that the adverse cardiovascular outcomes with smoking are real and it refutes "smoking paradox" theory very well and any other earlier investigations claiming lack of evidence for association between smoking intensity, duration and incident HF. It provides detailed objective evidence for association between pack-years, intensity and duration of smoking and both the phenotypes of HF.

While the association of smoking with HFrEF is explainable, how the smoking causes HFpEF is not clear. The investigators suggest several plausible mechanisms, including associated high blood pressure, increased oxidative stress, inflammation and mitochondrial dysfunction, all culminating into LV wall stiffness and remodeling.

Despite its many credentials, this ARIC substudy lacked in some aspects. It relied on self-reported smoking habit data, included subjects with history of coronary artery disease, did not measure systolic function in several individuals, and excluded relevant biomarkers such as C-reactive protein, troponin, and natriuretic peptides.

■ KEY PERSPECTIVE

The study has clear message to the public, health professionals, and policy makers that "smoking is injurious to health", backing up this statement with large body of evidence.[1] This becomes more relevant for HFpEF cohort as there we have limited management options and abstaining from smoking can be one such measure.

ARTICLE 2

Natural History and Prognostic Significance of Iron Deficiency and Anemia in Ambulatory Patients with Chronic Heart Failure

Graham FJ, Masini G, Pellicori P, Cleland JGF, Greenlaw N, Friday J, et al. Natural History and Prognostic Significance of Iron Deficiency and Anaemia in Ambulatory Patients with Chronic Heart Failure.
Eur J Heart Fail. 2022;24(5):807-17.

Abstract

Aims: Limited knowledge is available about the iron deficiency (ID) and anemia condition which are common in heart failure.

Methods and results: In this study investigation of prevalence, incidence and resolution of ID and anemia in a total of 906 enrolled patients with chronic heart failure [median age 73 (65–79) years, 70% men, 51% with heart failure with reduced ejection fraction] 1 year apart were done. When serum iron level noted ≤13 μmol/L in patients, ID and anemia were confirmed, as hemoglobin <13.0 g/dL for men or <12.0 g/dL for women. Also, considered FAIR-HF criteria for ID. Anemia without ID in 10%, ID without anemia in 23%, in 20% both, and in 47% neither found at baseline. Over 1-year percentages changed, but 157 (30%) patients had new-onset of ID, 104 (16%) new-onset anemia, while ID determined in 173 (44%) and anemia in 63 (23%). In multivariable models ($p = 0.02$) who remained iron replete (iron > 13 μmol/L), compared to those at 1-year mortality was higher in those with persistent or incident ID [hazard ratio (HR) 1.81 (1.23–2.67), and HR 1.40 (0.91–2.14), respectively]. Resolution of ID was associated with a lower mortality [HR 0.61 (0.44–0.86); $p = 0.004$] when compared to persistent ID. Changes in ID defined by FAIR-HF

(Ferinject Assessment in patients with IRon deficiency and chronic Heart Failure) criteria were not similarly associated with mortality. Even if anemia resolved, it was associated with a poor outcome.

Conclusion: In chronic heart failure, the prevalence and incidence of ID and anemia are high but it depends on the rate of resolution. A serum iron ≤13 µmol/L defined as persistent or incident ID and associated with higher mortality and resolution of ID with lower mortality.

ARTICLE COMMENTARY

Objective: To study the prevalence, incidence, and resolution of anemia and iron deficiency (ID) as variously defined, in chronic heart failure cohort.

Study design: It is an observational study enrolling patients from a single center clinic between 2002 and 2014, who had heart failure with reduced ejection fraction (HFrEF) [diagnosed as per the European Society of Cardiology (ESC) guidelines] and ID or anemia or both, following them at regular intervals for 5 years and their data was collected and analyzed.

Patients on erythropoietin analogs or IV iron therapy were excluded.

Other salient features/characteristics: A total number of 906 (33%) patients out of 2,763 patients were available for analysis in this study. As per the WHO criteria, anemia was defined as a hemoglobin of <12.0 g/dL in women and <13.0 g/dL in men. Iron indices studied included: serum ferritin, serum iron, transferrin, and transferrin saturation (TSAT). ID was defined as serum iron ≤13 µmol/L, in this study. The other criteria for ID, used in the FAIR-HF trial (adopted by the ESC), i.e., ferritin <100 µg/L or TSAT < 20% if ferritin 100–299 µg/L and TSAT of <20% alone, was also investigated in the study.

Result: At baseline, around 25% patients were neither suffering from anemia nor ID (defined as a serum iron ≤13 µmol/L). On follow-up at 1 year, among these, 22% developed ID alone, 8% ID and anemia, and 7% anemia only.

Among those 517, who were iron replete (i.e., ID absent irrespective of anemia status) at baseline, ID developed in 30% at 1 year, which was similar between those with HFrEF, heart failure with mid-range ejection fraction (HFmrEF), or heart failure with preserved ejection fraction (HFpEF). In multivariable analyses, only lower serum iron, lower hemoglobin and higher high-sensitivity C-reactive protein (hs-CRP) were significantly associated with incidence of ID.

Further, ID (based on serum iron criteria) resolved in 44% of the 389 ID patients at baseline, however, only 4% of these oral iron therapy. Resolution of ID was more likely in the absence of anemia at baseline.

Among 634 patients who were not anemic at baseline, 16% developed anemia at 1 year, which was similar for different strata of patients with HFrEF. Multivariable analyses revealed that increasing age and lower hemoglobin were strongly associated with incidence of anemia.

Among 272 anemic patients at the baseline, anemia resolved in 23%. Among these 68% had ID at baseline which persisted in 49% at 1 year.

Within 5 years, 30% patients died: 58% from cardiovascular (CV) causes, 39% from non-CV causes, and 3% from uncertain causes. Univariate analysis revealed that higher serum iron measured at 1 year had better subsequent survival, although the multivariable model did not show this benefit. Patients with persistent ID had the highest all-cause mortality [2.37 (1.76–3.20); $p<0.001$]. The survival benefit in relation to ID persisted even after multivariate analysis.

■ INTERPRETATION

This study systematically followed the natural history of anemia and iron deficiency in heart failure patient's cohort. The study utilized novel serum iron ≤ 13 µmol/L criteria to define iron deficiency and WHO criteria to define anemia. The recent ESC guidelines recommended criteria of ID based on FAIR-HF trial, failed to provide any clinically relevant patterns of prevalence, incidence, and resolution of ID. Applying the FAIR-HF criteria for ID, incidence among iron repletes, the resolution and persistence among ID, all were reported overtly compared to serum iron ≤ 13 µmol/L.

The study also studied patterns of prevalence, development, and resolution of ID with TSAT and showed resemblance in pattern with ID defined by serum iron criteria.

It seems fair to say to that serum iron criteria performed better for following the natural course of ID among all strata of HFrEF patients. However, survival benefit depicted in this study is still extrapolating too much if we say this benefit can only be seen with serum iron criteria only and not with TSAT or FAIR-HF criteria. This points to the fact that there are numerous clinical variables confounding the natural course and clinical outcomes in these HFrEF patients and may be serum iron criteria is less affected by them than the FAIR-HF criteria or TSAT criteria. But, even serum iron criteria failed to show this benefit after the multivariate adjustment. Nevertheless, this study also gives predictors of ID at 1 year like a lower serum iron or hemoglobin, reflecting borderline iron repletion, and higher hsCRP.

Further, it also emphasized the importance of treating anemia in heart failure patients.

■ KEY PERSPECTIVE

Most patients with heart failure have underlying comorbidities and they have or will develop ID and subsequently anemia also. Patients with persistent ID and anemia both may have a worse outcome compared to those in whom it resolves. The novel serum iron ≤13 µmol/L is more strongly associated with natural course of ID than that by the FAIR-HF criteria.[2]

ARTICLE 3

Impact of Moderate Aortic Stenosis in Patients with Heart Failure with Reduced Ejection Fraction

Khan KR, Khan OA, Chen C, Liu Y, Kandanelly RR, Jamiel PJ, et al. Impact of Moderate Aortic Stenosis in Patients With Heart Failure with Reduced Ejection Fraction.
J Am Coll Cardiol. 2023;81(13):1235-44.

Abstract

Background: Adverse outcomes in heart failure patients with reduced ejection fraction (HFrEF) are because of afterload from moderate aortic stenosis (AS).

Objectives: In this present study, authors assessed the clinical outcomes in HFrEF patients and moderate AS relative to those without AS and with severe AS.

Methods: HFrEF patients, defined by left ventricular ejection fraction (LVEF) < 50%, were not retrospectively identified as moderate or severe AS. All-cause mortality and heart failure (HF) hospitalization are the primary endpoints of study and was compared between groups and within a propensity score-matched cohort.

Results: In this study 9,133 patients with HFrEF were included, of whom 374 and 362 had moderate and severe AS, respectively. After average follow-up time of 3.1 years, the primary outcome observed in 62.7% of moderate AS patients versus 45.9% with no AS ($p < 0.0001$); similar rates in severe and moderate AS (62.0% vs. 62.7%; $p = 0.68$). Lower incidences of HF hospitalization (36.2% vs. 43.6%; $p < 0.05$) were noted in patients with severe AS and were expected to undergo aortic valve replacement (AVR) within the follow-up period. Moderate AS was found to be associated with an increased risk of HF hospitalization and mortality (HR 1.24; 95% CI 1.04–1.49; $p = 0.01$) within a propensity score-matched cohort and fewer days alive outside of the hospital ($p < 0.0001$). AVR was associated with improved survival (HR 0.60; 95% CI 0.36–0.99; $p < 0.05$).

Conclusion: Moderate AS is associated with increased rates of HF hospitalization and mortality in patients with HFrEF. More research is required in future to determine whether AVR in present population improves clinical outcomes or not.

ARTICLE COMMENTARY

Objective: To study the impact of moderate aortic stenosis (AS) on clinical outcomes in patients with heart failure with reduced ejection fraction (HFrEF) in comparison to those with no AS and severe AS.

Study design: It is a retrospective study based on echocardiographic database from Mass General Brigham Research Patient Data Registry, between 2016 and 2021. It identified patients with HFrEF, having left ventricle ejection fraction (LVEF) <50%, along with moderate AS. Further, two more groups were included, one with HFrEF and no AS (as negative control) and other with HFrEF with severe AS (as positive controls). Using propensity score matching, each of the 374 patients of HFrEF with moderate AS, was matched 1:1 to HFrEF patient with no AS.

Other salient features/characteristics: The three groups were compared in terms of primary and secondary outcomes during a follow-up of 3.1 years. The primary outcome was composite of heart failure (HF) hospitalization and mortality. Secondary outcomes included death, HF hospitalization, cumulative number of HF hospitalization and days alive out of the hospital (DAOH).

Results: The primary outcome rate was similar between HFrEF with moderate and severe AS, but it was much higher than in patients with HFrEF and no AS. All-cause mortality and DAOH also followed the same trend.

Heart failure hospitalization was significantly more with moderate AS compared to no AS group and there was trend toward significance for greater HF hospitalization with moderate AS compared to severe AS. This was without censoring for AVR.

With propensity-score matching, the significant differences in clinical outcomes persisted and even after multivariable adjustment, moderate AS remained independent predictor poorer outcomes.

■ INTERPRETATION

This study depicts how the moderate AS in HFrEF population affected the clinical course, indirectly proposing for early AVR in this cohort, but the evidence presented was weak. Despite propensity score matching, there were confounders in moderate and severe AS cohorts such as diabetes, atrial fibrillation, chronic kidney disease, coronary artery disease, altering the clinical outcomes. During the study, 12.2% in moderate AS group and 33.7% in severe AS group, underwent AVR. At that time, 80% of moderate AS group patients had progressed to severe AS. The early time to AVR in severe AS group (74 days) compared to moderate AS group (nearly 1 year) explains the higher incidence of HF hospitalization in the latter.

The grave course with moderate AS presented in this study is not new. In the past, we had reviews and meta-analysis suggesting the same. Similarly, the risk versus benefit of early intervention in moderate AS group has also been previously explored and early AVR is suggested to have improved survival.[3] Perhaps, a further investigation into subselecting high-risk cohort may help, as suggested by study of Ito et al., where LVEF deterioration began before AS became severe in those with an LVEF < 50%. Their study raised questions regarding the timing of intervention in such patients.[4]

■ CONCLUSION

This study suggests that moderate AS in HFrEF population increases the risk for adverse clinical outcomes and they may have better clinical course with early AVR. The evidence presented here, although not strong, but is enough to pave way for a large randomized control trial, which can answer this question better. It would be wise to wait for results from ongoing randomized clinical trials for AVR in moderate AS, before we finally conclude on this matter.

ARTICLE 4

Cardiogenic Shock from Heart Failure versus Acute Myocardial Infarction: Clinical Characteristics, Hospital Course, and 1-year Outcomes

Sinha SS, Rosner CM, Tehrani BN, Maini A, Truesdell AG, Lee SB, et al. Cardiogenic Shock From Heart Failure Versus Acute Myocardial Infarction: Clinical Characteristics, Hospital Course, and 1-Year Outcomes.
Circ Heart Fail. 2022;15(6):e009279.

Abstract

Background: Limited knowledge is available for patients with cardiogenic shock (CS) from heart failure (HF-CS) about their clinical characteristics, hospital course, and longitudinal outcomes as compared to acute myocardial infarction-cardiogenic shock (AMI-CS).

Methods: In this present study, 1-year outcomes of 520 (219 AMI-CS and 301 HF-CS) consecutive patients with CS (1/3/2017–12/31/2019) were examined in-hospital, a single center registry.

Results: The HF-CS cohort was younger (58.5 vs. 65.6 years, $p < 0.01$), lower cardiac power output (CPO) was seen (0.64 vs. 0.77 W), and temporary mechanical circulatory support (tMCS) was 34.9% versus 76.3%, $p < 0.001$. The mean age was 61.5 ± 13.5 years, 71% were male, 22% were black, and 63% had chronic kidney disease. After discharge, 133 AMI-CS and 229 HF-CS patients required similar rates of 30-day readmission (19.5% vs. 24.5%, $p = 0.30$) and major adverse cardiac and cerebrovascular events (23.3% vs. 28.8%, $p = 0.45$). HF-CS patients required lower 1-year mortality ($n = 123$, 42.6%) when compared to the AMI-CS patients ($n = 110$, 52.9%, $p = 0.03$). Also, lower cumulative 1-year mortality was observed in HF-CS patients (log-rank test, $p = 0.04$).

Conclusion: In spite of lower CPO and higher PCWP, HF-CS patients were younger, and, less likely to receive vasopressors or tMCS. Though HF-CS patients showed lower in-hospital and 1-year mortality, but both cohorts observed with similarly high rates of postdischarge major adverse cardiovascular and cerebrovascular events (MACCE) and 30-day readmission, emphasizing that both cohorts required careful long-term follow-up.

ARTICLE COMMENTARY

Objective: The main objective of the study is to compare hemodynamic presentations, treatment strategies and mortality outcomes among patients of cardiogenic shock due to heart failure (HF-CS) and acute myocardial infarction related cardiogenic shock (AMI-CS).[5]

Study design: This was a single center Virginia, US-based observational study enrolling patients diagnosed with CS based on criteria defined in SHOCK (SHould we emergently revascularize Occluded coronaries for Cardiogenic shocK) trial, i.e., systolic blood pressure (SBP) <90 mm Hg and cardiac index (CI) less than to 1.8 L/min/m^2 without vasopressors or 2.2 L/min/m^2 with vasopressors and a pulmonary capillary wedge pressure (PCWP) >15 mm Hg. Patients with CS of etiology other than AMI or heart failure (HF) were excluded.

Other salient features/characteristics: The data was retrospectively collected from national registries that included 30-day, 6-month, 1-year mortality, postdischarge hospitalization and any major adverse cardiovascular and cerebrovascular events (MACCE). Other relevant variables related to complications, use of mechanical circulatory support, were also determined. The patients were classified as per the Society for Cardiovascular Angiography and Interventions (SCAI) CS stage and CardShock risk scores and Inova Heart and Vascular Institute (IHVI) risk scores were also estimated.

The primary outcome was cumulative mortality at 1 year. The secondary endpoints were in-hospital mortality, 30-day hospital readmission, and MACCE within 1 year of hospital discharge.

Result: HF-CS cohort when compared to AMI-CS cohort had relatively younger population (58.5 vs. 65.6 years, $p < 0.001$), lesser number of cardiac arrest (15.9% vs. 35.2%, $p < 0.001$), lesser usage of vasopressor support (61.8% vs. 82.2%, $p < 0.001$), more impaired CPO (0.64 vs. 0.77 W, $p < 0.01$) and more elevated PCWP (25.4 vs. 22.2 mm Hg, $p < 0.001$).

Further HF-CS had significantly lower CardShock and IHVI Shock scores, but SCAI shock stages were similar between the two cohorts.

The HF-CS patients were also less likely to receive any temporary mechanical circulatory support (tMCS) devices. Instead, they were more likely to receive long-term advanced HF therapies, including durable ventricular assist device (VAD) and heart transplantation. HF-CS patients experienced lower rates of complications, but had a longer hospital stay.

In-hospital mortality and cardiac causes of mortality were both significantly lower for HF-CS compared to AMI-CS. Among those who survived to hospital discharge, HF-CS cohort had higher episodes of acute decompensated HF. However, AMI-CS patients were more likely to experience recurrent AMI.

In the AMI-CS group, SCAI stage D or E, diabetes mellitus, age, and cardiac arrest were independently associated with 1-year mortality. In the HF-CS group, besides above-mentioned factors, index GFR < 60 mL/min was also an independent predictor of 1-year mortality.

■ INTERPRETATION

This study establishes HF-CS and AMI-CS as different phenotypic entities. AMI-CS cohort, which was also the older cohort, showed hemodynamic derangements that were relatively less adapted, resulting in higher CardShock and IHVI scores despite having higher CPO and lower PCWP. This explains their need for higher vasopressor and MCS requirements and higher rates of in-hospital cardiac arrest, mortality, MACCE, and complications and on follow-up higher recurrence rate of myocardial infarction (MI). These features are quite distinct from those of HF-CS cohort. HF-CS phenotype represented an acute on chronic phenomenon with better chronic compensation. They had settled at lower CPO and higher PCWP, lesser end-organ hypoperfusion, malignant arrhythmias, and this translated into lower in-hospital mortality, lesser requirement of vasopressors and MCS, but advanced HF therapies like durable VAD and heart transplantation were more frequently used with HF-CS patients. Both AMI-CS and HF-CS had high 30-day recurrent hospitalization and majority were due to acute HF. This supports the fact that vigilant postdischarge clinical follow-up particularly in first month, can prevent such event. Further observations from the study reveals that HF-CS group is more vulnerable for mortality during posthospital discharge phase and survival beyond this point represents an important milestone in overall trajectory of these patients.

The study had a few limitations like it was a single center study and no specific threshold for use and timing of temporary MCS was defined. Further, there was no differentiation into acute versus acute on chronic heart failure and data on usage of guideline directed medical therapy was missing.

■ KEY PERSPECTIVE

Significant differences were observed among the two cohorts of CS, namely AMI-CS and HF-CS, in terms of presentations, hemodynamic profiles, hospital outcomes and 1-year clinical outcomes. Further studies are required to better delineate these two subsets of CS and formulating necessary steps to improve the clinical outcomes.

REFERENCES

1. Lee H, Son YJ. Influence of Smoking Status on Risk of Incident Heart Failure: A Systematic Review and Meta-Analysis of Prospective Cohort Studies. Int J Environ Res Pub Health. 2019;16: 2697.
2. Anker SD, Comin Colet J, Filippatos G, Willenheimer R, Dickstein K, Drexler H et al; FAIR-HF Trial Investigators. Ferric carboxymaltose in patients with heart failure and iron deficiency. N Engl J Med. 2009;361(25):2436-48.
3. Coisne A, Scotti A, Latib A, Montaigne D, Ho EC, Ludwig S, et al. Impact of Moderate Aortic Stenosis on Long-Term Clinical Outcomes: A Systematic Review and Meta-Analysis. JACC Cardiovasc Interv. 2022;15(16):1664-74.
4. Ito S, Miranda WR, Nkomo VT, Connolly HM, Pislaru SV, Greason KL, et al. Reduced Left Ventricular Ejection Fraction in Patients With Aortic Stenosis. J Am Coll Cardiol. 2018;71(12):1313-21.
5. Hochman JS, Sleeper LA, Webb JG, Sanborn TA, White HD, Talley JD, et al. Early revascularization in acute myocardial infarction complicated by cardiogenic shock. SHOCK Investigators. Should We Emergently Revascularize Occluded Coronaries for Cardiogenic Shock. N Engl J Med. 1999;341(9):625-34.

SECTION 3

Imaging in Heart Failure

Section Editor: **MK Das**

Co-Editors: Shantanu Sengupta, Mona Bhatia

ARTICLE 1

Quantified Mitral Regurgitation and Left Atrial Function in Heart Failure with Reduced Ejection Fraction: Interplay and Outcome Implications

Malagoli A, Rossi L, Zanni A, Sticozzi C, Piepoli MF, Benfari G. Quantified mitral regurgitation and left atrial function in heart failure with reduced ejection fraction: interplay and outcome implications.
Eur J Heart Fail. 2022;24(4):694-702.

Abstract

Aims: In heart failure patients with reduced ejection fraction (HFrEF), the clinical and prognostic importance of functional mitral regurgitation (FMR) has been highly disputed. Present study in a prospective cohort of consecutive HFrEF outpatients, designed to explain FMR linkage to cardiovascular (CV) outcomes and the interplay with left atrial (LA) function.

Methods and results: A total number of 286 consecutive outpatients with chronic HFrEF were prospectively registered. FMR was quantification done by effective regurgitant orifice area (EROA). Measurement of global peak atrial longitudinal strain (PALS) was done by speckle tracking echocardiography. Congestive heart failure hospitalization and/or CV death are the primary endpoint outcomes. The primary endpoint occurred in 99 patients (35%) during a mean follow-up of 4.1 ± 1.5 years. The spline modeling of the risk by FMR severity showed an excess event risk starting at about the EROA value of 0.1 cm^2. Noticed a remarkable graded association between the EROA strata, even if tested per 0.1 cm^2 increase, and the risk of CV events [hazard ratio (HR) EROA per 0.10 cm^2 increase 1.42; 95% confidence interval (CI) 1.19–1.68; $p < 0.0001$]. Regardless of LA function (HR 2.34; 95% CI 1.29–4.19; $p = 0.005$) EROA ≥ 0.30 cm^2 was associated with CV events. Only in patients presented with reduced LA function (PALS < 14%) (5-year CV event rate 51 ± 4%), less severe FMR (EROA ≥ 0.10 cm^2) was associated with a dismal outcome; contrariwise, when preserved global PALS and FMR coexisted (5-year CV event rate 38 ± 6%) the risk of events was relatively reduced.

Conclusion: Results of present study upgraded the current knowledge on the independent association between FMR and CV outcome among HFrEF outpatients. LA function mitigates the clinical consequences of mitral regurgitation within a moderate EROA range, provided measurable proof of the interplay between regurgitation and LA compliance.

ARTICLE COMMENTARY

Editorial comments: Heart failure (HF) is a grave and global problem with frequent hospitalization and high 1-year (25%) and 5-year (50%) mortality despite guideline-directed medical therapy (GDMT).[1,2] The two articles, one by Malagoli et al.[3] and the second one by Inciardi et al.[4] reminded us all about the active role of the left atrium in influencing the natural history of heart failure.

In the first study, it is discussed that functional mitral regurgitation (FMR) caused by annular dilatation is a frequent accompaniment in HF. However, this is not well studied in terms of clear-cut therapeutic implications. In the second study, Inciardi et al. used simple measurement of left atrial (LA) diameter by transthoracic echocardiography (TTE) and demonstrated that the LA adverse remodeling (LAAR) over a period of time had the predictive capacity on the risk of primary endpoints namely composite of all-cause mortality and hospitalizations.

Both studies ignite the minds to evaluate the LA not only to predict the events in HFrEF but also to triage the patients for therapy. Malagoli et al. have done a good job in bringing out the role of regurgitant volume and vena contracta or effective regurgitant orifice area (EROA) as an independent link between FMR and subsequent survival. They also demonstrated that the spectrum of LA function quantified by speckle track echocardiography (STE) was not only reflective of the functional abnormality but also had the independent prognostic value in HF patients with reduced ejection fraction (HFrEF). On the other hand, Inciardi et al. attributed LAAR as a single test to prognosticate while following up on patients with heart failure.

Methodologies: The study by Malagoli et al. enrolled 402 patients of HFrEF < 40% in the age group of 18–85 years after optimizing the GDMT and followed them up prospectively for 6 months during 2011–2015 with exclusion criteria of atrial arrhythmias, primary valve disease, prosthetic valves, chronic obstructive pulmonary disease (COPD), chronic kidney disease (CKD), malignancy, refractory angina, admission for worsening of HF or after percutaneous coronary intervention (PCI) in last 3 months before enrollment.

After all the clinical data were recorded, the patients underwent transthoracic echocardiography (TTE) which measured left ventricular end-diastolic volume index (LVEDVi) and left ventricular end-systolic volumes (LVESD), LA volume, proximal iso-velocity surface area (PISA) and EROA as per standard protocol.

EROA ≥ 0.30 cm^2 was taken as the criteria for severe FMR.[5] STE ascertaining longitudinal strain curves for each atrial segment gave the idea of peak atrial longitudinal strain (PALS). During the same period, the plasma B-type natriuretic peptide levels were assayed, the range criteria being 10–5,000 pg/mL. The follow-up was done either during the clinic visit or transtelephonically. The primary endpoints were hospitalization for HF (HHF) or cardiovascular death occurring within 5 years of inclusion.

Ultimately 286 patients fulfilled the criteria for FMR. 46 patients (16%) could not be evaluated for further follow-up. LA enlargement was frequently found with LAVi max of 47 ± 16 mL/m^2. The median global PALS during LA systole was present in 17.7% (range 27–49.2%). STE was feasible in >95% segments and inter- and intraobserver variation for PALS was low. The primary endpoint occurred in 99 patients over a period of 4.1 ± 1.5 years and secondary endpoints in 80 patients with 92% deaths and 8% non-CV deaths.

The univariate Cox-regression analysis for 0.10 cm^2 EROA increase revealed a significant association of FMR with cardiac events with HR 2.20; 95% CI 1.40–3.46; $p = 0.0007$ in positive group and HR 1.42; 95% CI 1.19–1.68; $p < 0.0001$ in absent group.

In multivariate analysis adjusted for age, sex, LVEF and global PALS, EROA had independent predictive value for primary events (HR 1.23; 95% CI 1.01–1.48; $p = 0.04$). Though the correlation was modest, but similar results were also found with Global PALS when EROA was <0.10 cm^2. It was worth noting that these patient groups had fourfold increases in BNP value and higher NYHA class (III–IV); the higher EROA values correlated well with higher NYHA class and BNP level even after adjusting for CKD and LA function and had worse prognosis in HFrEF.

Inciardi et al. studied 632 patients with optimized GDMT for a period of 9 months. The LA dimension was assessed by measuring linear anterior-posterior dimensions of LA by TTE. LA adverse remodeling (LAAR) was defined as an increase in LA dimensions from the base level to a 9-month follow-up. LAAR was found in 247 patients (35%). The primary and secondary endpoints were evaluated after follow-up for a mean period of 13 months (8–18 months range). The uptitration of angiotensin-converting enzyme inhibitors (ACEIs)/angiotensin receptor blockers (ARBs) was done with a larger LA size and this lessened the LAAR and thus primary endpoints of a composite of all-cause mortality and hospitalizations. The multivariate analysis offered a number of variables to be predictors of LAAR. They were: (i) larger base-line LA diameter (OR 0.90; 95% CI 0,87–0.93; $p < 0.001$), (ii) higher ACEI/ARB fraction target dose at 3 months (OR 0.56; 95% CI 0.34–0.92; $p = 0.022$). They had a lower likelihood of LAAR which had an increased risk of a composite of all-cause mortality or HHF. The absence of a history of atrial fibrillation had a higher association with the variables and LAAR.

Strength and limitations of the studies: The first one was a single-center study with a relatively smaller sample size undergoing the same STE device used for LV, the composite primary endpoint had adequate power to predict the survival model and it is fair to recommend EROA, and STE along with other standard values and BNP measurements for prognostication of the patients with HFrEF. The second study, a post hoc analysis of a prospective study did not use a core laboratory and the inter- and intraobserver variability were not evaluated. Follow-up of 25% of patients limited the power to assess the efficacy of ACEI/ARB on LA enlargement. Only a small proportion of patients with heart failure with preserved ejection fraction (HFpEF) were included and thus no extrapolation was possible with the whole spectrum of heart failure. Besides the various functional assessment measures like volumetric measurement and STE were not done thus exposing the limitations of the study.

Conclusion: LA is not just a bystander but an active functional part of the heart. When there is FMR, the various studied parameters like EROA and STE influence the morbidity, HHF, and mortality in patients of HFrEF. The LAAR, on the other hand, also gives some hints about the prognosis of the patients of heart failure. However, larger studies are warranted to definitely conclude the implications of LA in the overall follow-up and prognosis of the patients.

ARTICLE 2

Clinical Implications of Left Atrial Changes after Optimization of Medical Therapy in Patients with Heart Failure

Inciardi RM, Pagnesi M, Lombardi CM, Anker SD, Cleland JG, Dickstein K, et al. Clinical implications of left atrial changes after optimization of medical therapy in patients with heart failure.
Eur J Heart Fail. 2022;24(11):2131-9.

Abstract

Aims: Less is known about the prognostic relevance of changes in left atrial (LA) dimensions in heart failure (HF) patients. Present study evaluated changes in LA dimension and their relation with outcomes after optimization of guideline-directed medical therapy (GDMT) in new-onset or worsening HF in patients.

Methods and results: In 632 patients (mean age 65.8 ± 12.1 years, 22.3% female) enrolled in BIOSTAT-CHF LA diameter was measured at baseline and 9 months after GDMT optimization. An increase in LA diameter on transthoracic echocardiography between baseline and 9 months is stated as LA adverse remodeling (LAAR). Patients were followed for a median of 13 further months after the 9-month visit. In 247 patients (39%), LAAR was observed. An independent association was observed for larger baseline LA diameter [odds ratio (OR) 0.90; 95% confidence interval (CI) 0.87–0.93; $p < 0.001$] and uptitration to higher doses of angiotensin-converting enzyme inhibitors or angiotensin receptor blockers (ACEIs/ARBs) (OR 0.56; 95% CI 0.34–0.92; $p = 0.022$) with lower likelihood of LAAR. An association of LAAR with an increased risk of the composite of all-cause mortality or HF hospitalization (log-rank $p = 0.007$ and adjusted hazard ratio 1.73; 95% CI 1.22–2.45; $p = 0.002$) was observed. In patients without a history of atrial fibrillation (p for interaction = 0.009), the association was more noticeable.

Conclusion: LAAR was associated with an unfavorable outcome and was prevented by ACEI/ARB uptitration, among patients enrolled in BIOSTAT-CHF. Changes in LA dimension may be a useful marker of response to treatment and improve risk stratification in HF patients.

ARTICLE COMMENTARY

Please refer Article 1.

ARTICLE 3

Strain Echocardiography in Predicting LV Dysfunction in RV Apical Pacing

Datta G, Dastidar DG, Chakraborty H. Strain echocardiography in predicting LV dysfunction in RV apical pacing. *Indian Heart J. 2023;75(1):77-81.*

Abstract

Right ventricular (RV) pacing is associated with a reduction in left ventricular (LV) systolic function, thought to be mediated by pacing-induced ventricular dyssynchrony.

After RV pacing, the prevalence of heart failure is reported to range from 31 ± 3%. In present study, 60 subjects with high-grade atrioventricular block and complete heart block (CHB) were scheduled to undergo RV apical pacing. At baseline, 1 month and 12 months two-dimensional (2D) echocardiography was done. A reduction in LV ejection fraction (LVEF) to <45% is known as pacing-induced cardiomyopathy. Using all advanced software package [cardiac wall motion quantification (CMQ); Toshiba Medical Systems] strain was evaluated off-line from digitally stored images. For individual myocardial segments longitudinal strain was measured from the apical four-chamber, two-chamber, and long-axis views (16 segment AHA/ASE model). No one had shown LV dysfunction at baseline based on 2D and strain echocardiographic imaging. Consequently, at 1 month 18 patients were identified who to develop low global longitudinal strain (GLS) score (less than −14.5). All 18 patients developed LV dysfunction on 2D echocardiography on subsequent follow-up at 1 year. Hence, strain imaging with GLS score assisted in early recognition of LV dysfunction in RV apical pacing subjects. Significant association observed for pacing-induced cardiomyopathy with high-grade AV block with pacemaker dependency. But, no significant associations with other comorbidities such as diabetes, hypertension, and ischemic heart disease or with the type of medication intake were found. Conversely, there a statistically significant association with heart failure was found.

ARTICLE COMMENTARY

Right ventricular (RV) pacing is often associated with a reduction in left ventricular (LV) systolic function. The prevalence of heart failure (HF) after RV pacing is reported to range from 31 ± 3%. This study by Datta et al. evaluated the role of 2D strain imaging by echocardiography for prediction of LV dysfunction in patients undergoing RV pacing. For this, 60 patients were included in this investigator-initiated prospective observational cohort study. Patients had either high-grade atrioventricular block or complete heart block (CHB). All patients underwent detailed 2D echocardiography at baseline, 1 month, and 12 months. Pacing-induced LV dysfunction was defined as a reduction in LV ejection fraction (LVEF) to <45%. None had LV dysfunction at baseline based on 2D and strain echocardiographic imaging. Subsequently, 18 patients were detected to develop low global longitudinal strain (GLS) score (less than −14.5) at 1 month. On subsequent follow-up at 1 year, all 18 patients developed LV dysfunction on

2D echocardiography. Thus, strain imaging with GLS score helped in early detection of LV dysfunction in RV apical pacing subjects. Pacing-induced LV dysfunction had significant association with high-grade atrioventricular (AV) block with pacemaker dependency. It had no significant associations with other comorbidities such as diabetes, hypertension, ischemic heart disease or with the type of medication intake. However, there was a statistically significant association with heart failure.

ARTICLE 4

Left Ventricular Global Longitudinal Strain Imaging in Identifying Subclinical Myocardial Dysfunction Among COVID-19 Survivors

Kujur PP, Jhala M, Bhondve A, Lanjewar C, Matta R, Deshmukh H. Left ventricular global longitudinal strain imaging in identifying subclinical myocardial dysfunction among COVID-19 survivors.
Indian Heart J. 2022;74(1):51-5.

Abstract

Background: Severe acute respiratory syndrome-related coronavirus 2 (SARS-CoV-2) virus causes a multisystem viral infection known as "coronavirus disease 2019 (COVID-19)". The disease also presented variety of cardiovascular manifestations contributing to morbidity as well as mortality, apart from acute severe respiratory illness which causes high mortality. After the COVID-19 pandemic, evident from multiple studies showed that cardiac dysfunction and myocarditis are well-known complications of COVID-19. Conversely, no studies adequately conducted in Indian patients either by echocardiography or by any other imaging modalities like cardiac magnetic resonance imaging (MRI).

Methodology: In COVID-19, survivors present study analyzed the severity of left ventricular (LV) dysfunction. After 1 month of discharge, a total of 100 patients of COVID-19 who had no underlying cardiovascular diseases underwent echocardiography and global longitudinal strain (GLS) imaging was included. In this study, cohort patients with mild 42 (42%), moderate 46 (46%), and severe 12 (12%) COVID-19 disease as defined by computed tomography (CT) severity score were enrolled.

Results: Here, in this study, we noted that total 36 (36%) patients had reduced ejection fraction (EF) which included 11 patients having EF < 40% and remaining 25 (25%) having EF 40–50% ($p < 0.002$). Abnormal GLS values with normal EF which is suggestive of subclinical myocarditis observed in 22 (22%) patients. In 7 (19.5%) patients who had severe COVID-19, LV dysfunction was observed while in 29 (80.5%) noncritical patients mild to moderate LV dysfunction observed.

Conclusion: Present study illustrated that myocardial dysfunction is common in COVID-19 regardless of disease severity. Among these patients, 2D-echocardiography with GLS is likely to detect early LV dysfunction.

ARTICLE COMMENTARY

Coronavirus disease 2019 (COVID-19) infection is a multisystem viral infection caused by severe acute respiratory syndrome-related coronavirus 2 (SARS-CoV-2) virus. This has also been known to affect the heart contributing to morbidity as well as mortality. Cardiac dysfunction and myocarditis are well established complications of COVID-19 as evident in multiple studies after the COVID-19 pandemic. This study by Kujur et al. highlighted the effect of COVID-19 on heart as assessed by left ventricular global longitudinal strain (LVGLS) in Indian patients 100 consecutive patients of COVID-19 after 1 month of discharge who had no underlying cardiovascular diseases underwent echocardiography and global longitudinal strain (GLS) imaging. This study cohort included patients with mild 42 (42%), moderate 46 (46%), and severe 12 (12%). COVID-19 disease as defined by computed tomography (CT) severity score. The study revealed observed 36 (36%) patients had reduced ejection fraction (EF) which included 11 patients having EF < 40% and remaining 25 (25%) having EF 40–50% ($p < 0.002$). 22 (22%) patients had abnormal LVGLS values with normal ejection fraction. LV dysfunction was seen in 7 (19.5%) patients who had severe COVID-19 while mild to moderate LV dysfunction observed in 29 (80.5%) noncritical patients. This study demonstrated that LV dysfunction is common in COVID-19 regardless of disease severity and can be picked up by 2D-echocardiography with LVGLS assessment.

ARTICLE 5

Prognostic Value of Global Longitudinal Strain in Patients with Heart Failure with Improved Ejection Fraction

Janwanishstaporn S, Cho JY, Feng S, Brann A, Seo JS, Narezkina A, et al. Prognostic Value of Global Longitudinal Strain in Patients With Heart Failure With Improved Ejection Fraction.
JACC Heart Fail. 2022;10(1):27-37.

Abstract

Objectives: The present study aimed to determine association of global longitudinal strain (GLS) is with the natural history of patients with heart failure with improved ejection fraction (HFimpEF).

Background: In patients heart failure with reduced EF, left ventricular ejection fraction (LVEF) often improves. However, variability in the clinical course of patients with HFimpEF was noticed. A sensitive indicator of LV systolic function, i.e., GLS could help in predicting risk of future events in this population.

Methods: This is a retrospective analysis of HF patients presented with LVEF > 40% on index echocardiogram who had shown LVEF < 40% on initial study and improvement of ≥10%. By two-dimensional speckle-tracking software on index echocardiography GLS was assessed. Primary endpoints were time of first occurrence of cardiovascular mortality or HF hospitalization/emergency treatment.

Results: Of the total 289 HFimpEF patients, median absolute values of GLS (aGLS) and LVEF from index echocardiography were 12.7% (IQR 10.8–14.7%) and 52% (IQR 46–58%), respectively. The primary endpoint occurred less frequently in patients with aGLS above the median than below it (21% vs. 34%; $p = 0.014$); HR 0.51; 95% CI 0.33–0.81; $p = 0.004$ over 53 months following index echocardiography. Each 1% increase in a GLS on index echocardiogram was associated with a lower likelihood of the composite endpoint when considered as a continuous variable; HR 0.86; 95% CI 0.79–0.93; $p < 0.001$, after multivariable adjustment an association persisted; HR 0.90; 95% CI 0.82–0.97; $p = 0.01$. Observed the association of lower aGLS with increased likelihood of deterioration in LVEF.

Conclusion: GLS is a strong predictor for future HF events and deterioration in cardiac function in HFimpEF patients.

ARTICLE COMMENTARY

Left ventricular (LV) ejection fraction (EF) is known to improve in patients with heart failure with reduced EF (HFrEF). There has been a lot of interests in knowing the clinical course of patients with HFimpEF. LV global longitudinal strain (GLS) is a marker of LV systolic function and can help to predict risk of future events in this population apart from LVEF. In this single center, retrospective, cohort observational study by Janwanishstaporn S et al., 289 patients were included. The analysis was done of HF patients with LVEF > 40% on index echocardiogram who had LVEF < 40% on initial study and improvement of >10%. LVGLS was assessed by two-dimensional speckle-tracking software on index echocardiography. Primary outcome was defined as time to first occurrence of cardiovascular mortality or HF hospitalization/emergency treatment. The median GLS and LVEF from index echocardiography were −12.7% (IQR 10.8–14.7%) and 52% (IQR 46–58%), respectively. Over 53 months following index echocardiography, the primary endpoint occurred less frequently in patients with GLS above the median than below it (21% vs. 34%; $p = 0.014$); HR 0.51; 95% CI 0.33–0.81; $p = 0.004$. Each 1% increase in GLS on index echocardiogram was associated with a lower likelihood of the composite endpoint; HR 0.86; 95% CI 0.79–0.93; $p < 0.001$. Also, lower GLS was associated with increased likelihood of deterioration in LVEF. So, this study concluded that in patients with HFimpEF, GLS is a strong predictor for future HF events and deterioration in cardiac function.

ARTICLE 6

Right Ventricular Dysfunction in Patients with New-onset Heart Failure: Longitudinal Follow-up during Guideline-directed Medical Therapy

Ansari Ramandi MM, van Melle JP, Gorter TM, Hoendermis ES, van Veldhuisen DJ, Nauta JF, et al. Right ventricular dysfunction in patients with new-onset heart failure: longitudinal follow-up during guideline-directed medical therapy. *Eur J Heart Fail.* 2022;24(12):2226-34.

Abstract

Aims: In heart failure (HF) patients, improvement in left ventricular ejection fraction (LVEF) after uptitration of guideline-directed medical therapy (GDMT) has been well described. Limited data is available about the prevalence and clinical course of right ventricular dysfunction (RVD) in patients with new-onset of HF.

Methods and results: A total of 625 patients with a recent (<3 months) diagnosis of HF were referred to a specialized nurse-led HF clinic for protocolized uptitration of GDMT from 2012 to 2018. At the follow-up visit, tricuspid annular plane systolic excursion (TAPSE) <17 mm, i.e., RVD was assessed at baseline. For a mean of 3.3 ± 1.9 years patients were followed for the combined endpoint of all-cause mortality and HF hospitalization. Out of the 625 patients, 241 (38.6%) patients showed RVD at baseline. Patients with RVD were older, more symptomatic, had a lower LVEF, and more often had a history of cardiothoracic surgery and atrial fibrillation. Right ventricular function normalized in 49% of the patients with baseline RVD, after average follow-up of 9 months. Here, observed an association of RVD at baseline with a higher risk of the combined endpoint [hazard ratio (HR) 1.62; 95% confidence interval (CI) 1.21–2.18]. Independent of baseline TAPSE, age, sex, and LVEF, right ventricular function normalization was associated with a lower risk for the combined endpoint (HR 0.56; 95% CI 0.31–0.99).

Conclusion: It was concluded from this study that more than one-third of patients with new-onset of HF have RVD. Also, observed association of RVD with a higher risk of all-cause mortality and HF hospitalization. Recovery of RVD regularly occurs during uptitration of GDMT and observed to be is associated with improved clinical outcomes.

ARTICLE COMMENTARY

The study by Ramadi et al. was a retrospective longitudinal cohort follow-up study. About 625 consecutive patients with a diagnosis of new-onset heart failure (HF) were included from a nurse-led HF clinic for protocolized uptitration of guideline-directed medical management (GDMT) based on the guidelines of HF from the European Society of Cardiology. The follow-up visit was at 9 months or the closest visit to make sure that medications were fully uptitrated. Right ventricular dysfunction (RVD) was defined as tricuspid annular plane systolic excursion (TAPSE) <17 mm and was assessed at baseline and at follow-up visit. Follow-up was for combined endpoint of all-cause mortality and HF hospitalization for a mean of 3.3 ± 1.9 years. Of the 625 patients, 241 (38.6%) patients had RVD at baseline. Patients with RVD were older, more symptomatic, had a lower LVEF, and more often had a history of cardiothoracic surgery and atrial fibrillation. After a median follow-up of 9 months, RV function recovered and normalized in 49% of the patients with baseline RVD. RVD at baseline was associated with a higher risk of the combined endpoint [hazard ratio (HR) 1.62; 95% confidence interval (CI) 1.21–2.18]. RV function normalization was associated with a lower risk for the combined endpoint (HR 0.56; 95% CI 0.31–0.99), independent of baseline TAPSE, age, sex, and LVEF. So, this study concluded that around 38% patients with new-onset of HF have RVD. RVD is associated with a higher risk of all-cause mortality and HF hospitalization. Uptitration of GDMT helps in recovery of RVD and is associated with improved clinical outcomes.

ARTICLE 7

Correlation of Serum ST2 Levels with Severity of Diastolic Dysfunction on Echocardiography and Findings on Cardiac MRI in Patients with Heart Failure with Preserved Ejection Fraction

Agrawal V, Hardas S, Gujar H, Phalgune DS. Correlation of serum ST2 levels with severity of diastolic dysfunction on echocardiography and findings on cardiac MRI in patients with heart failure with preserved ejection fraction. *Indian Heart J. 2022;74(3):229-34.*

Abstract

Objective: The purpose of the present study was to discover a correlation of serum suppression of tumorigenicity 2 (ST2) levels with severity of diastolic dysfunction on echocardiography and cardiac magnetic resonance imaging (CMRI) in patients with heart failure preserved ejection fraction (HFpEF).

Methods: In present study, 50 patients fulfilling diagnostic criteria for HFpEF and aged ≥18 years were included. For all patients performed ST2 levels, two-dimensional (2D) echocardiography and CMRI. Noted the important parameter such as left ventricular ejection fraction, E/A, septal E/E', left atrial volume index (LAVI), tricuspid regurgitation (TR), assessment of diastolic dysfunction, T1 mapping in milliseconds, and late gadolinium enhancement (LGE) in percentage. The primary outcome endpoint was to know the correlation of ST2 levels with severity of diastolic dysfunction, while the secondary endpoints were to rule out correlation of ST2 levels with native T1 mapping and LGE on CMRI.

Results: A statistically significant and positive correlation with E/E' ($r = 0.837$), peak TR velocity ($r = 0.373$), LAVI ($r = 0.74$), E/A ($r = 0.420$), and T1 values in milliseconds ($r = 0.619$) showed by ST2 levels. Between ST2 level and LGE in % ($r = 0.145$) they have not noticed any statistically significant correlation. The mean ST2 levels in patients with E/E' > 14 and E/E'< 14 were 110.8 and 36.1, respectively ($p < 0.05$). In patients who had diastolic dysfunction grade III (126.4) and New York Heart Association class IV (133.3) the mean ST2 levels were significantly higher.

Conclusion: To provide the best care and the diagnosis of left ventricular diastolic dysfunction in HFpEF patients evaluation of ST2 adds significant knowledge.

ARTICLE COMMENTARY

The global prevalence of heart failure is rapidly increasing, with high hospitalization and mortality rates. Heart failure patients can be categorized based on ejection fraction. Heart failure with preserved ejection fraction (HFpEF) has a high mortality rate and debilitating symptoms. Biomarkers like B-type natriuretic peptide (BNP) and N-terminal pro B-type natriuretic peptide (NT-proBNP) are used for diagnosis and prognosis. Myocardial fibrosis is a key factor in HFpEF development and cardiac MRI parameters like LGE and T1 relaxation time are being studied. There is limited research on biomarkers and imaging findings in HFpEF patients. This study aimed to correlate serum ST2 levels with diastolic dysfunction severity on echocardiography and cardiac magnetic resonance imaging (CMRI) in HFpEF patients.

A prospective observational study conducted in Pune (Poona Hospital and Research Center), India, aimed to investigate the correlation between ST2 levels and the severity of diastolic dysfunction in patients with heart failure with preserved ejection fraction (HFpEF). The study included patients over 18 years of age who met the diagnostic criteria for HFpEF. Patients with certain chronic inflammatory conditions were excluded. The study assessed ST2 levels using a monoclonal lateral flow immunoassay and performed various tests, including echocardiography and CMRI, to evaluate cardiac function and fibrosis. Echocardiography assessment included estimation of left ventricular ejection fraction (LVEF), diastolic function parameters (E/A, septal E/E'), left atrial volume, left atrial volume index (LAVI), and tricuspid regurgitation (TR) systolic jet velocity to evaluate diastolic dysfunction severity. The primary objective was to examine the correlation between ST2 levels and diastolic dysfunction severity, while secondary objectives focused on the correlation with native T1 mapping and late gadolinium enhancement (LGE) on CMRI. The study calculated the sample size based on a specific formula (sample size – 42) and used statistical analyses such as Fisher's exact test, Mann–Whitney U test, and Pearson's correlation coefficient to analyze the data. The significance level was set at 0.05.

ST2 levels were significantly higher in patients with diastolic dysfunction grade III compared to grades I and II. Median ST2 levels were 110.8 in patients with E/E' > 14 and 36.1 in patients with E/E' ≤ 14. Mean ST2 levels were significantly higher in NYHA class III and IV compared to class I and II. There was a significant correlation between ST2 levels and E/E0, peak TR velocity, LAVI, and E/A, with increasing ST2 levels associated with higher values in these parameters. The difference in ST2 levels was statistically significant based on the grade of diastolic dysfunction. Additionally, a higher percentage of patients with diastolic dysfunction grade III had ST2 levels >35 U/mL. There was a statistically significant positive correlation between ST2 levels and T1 values (in milliseconds) ($p < 0.001$, $r = 0.619$). As ST2 levels increased, T1 values also increased. In a considerable portion of the sample, no statistically significant correlation ($p = 0.125$, $r = 0.145$) was observed between ST2 levels and LGE.

Previous studies have shown a correlation between soluble ST2 (sST2) and left ventricular mass index with native T1 mapping in dilated cardiomyopathy patients. In this study on HFpEF patients, a significant positive correlation ($r = 0.619$) was found between ST2 levels and T1 mapping (in milliseconds) on CMRI. However, there was no significant correlation between ST2 and LGE on CMRI, consistent with other studies where the correlation was weak ($r = 0.130$, $p = 0.32$). This highlights the potential of using T1 mapping as an imaging marker for myocardial fibrosis, but further research is needed to understand the relationship between ST2 and LGE in HFpEF patients.

The highlight of this study is the unique attempt to find an association between serum ST2 levels and native T1 mapping in HFpEF patients. Limitations included small sample size, single center design, lack of control group, and no NT-proBNP/BNP measurements. Findings are hypothesis-generating and require confirmation in larger populations.

Echocardiography is known to assess diastolic function, while studies have compared serum ST2 levels with clinical and echocardiographic parameters in HFpEF. However, limited studies have explored the correlation between serum ST2 levels and CMRI parameters (T1 mapping and LGE) in HFpEF patients. This research has investigated the correlation between ST2, T1 mapping, and LGE, which has not been previously studied and delivered some encouraging results.

ARTICLE 8

Artificial Intelligence for Contrast-free MRI: Scar Assessment in Myocardial Infarction using Deep Learning-based Virtual Native Enhancement

Zhang Q, Burrage MK, Shanmuganathan M, Gonzales RA, Lukaschuk E, Thomas KE, et al. Artificial Intelligence for Contrast-Free MRI: Scar Assessment in Myocardial Infarction Using Deep Learning-Based Virtual Native Enhancement. Circulation. 2022;146(20):1492-503.

Abstract

Background: Using cardiovascular magnetic resonance late gadolinium enhancement (LGE) myocardial scars are assessed noninvasively as an imaging gold standard. Many advantages were provided by contrast-free approach, includes a quicker and low-cost scan without contrast-associated problems.

Methods: A novel technology is virtual native enhancement (VNE) can produce virtual LGE-like images without the need for contrast. VNE combines cine imaging and native T1 maps to produce LGE-like images using artificial intelligence VNE was developed for patients with previous myocardial infarction from 4271 data sets (912 patients); each data set comprises slice position-matched cine, T1 maps, and LGE images. After quality control, 3002 data sets (775 patients) were used for development and 291 data sets (68 patients) for testing. The VNE generator was trained using generative adversarial networks, using 2 adversarial discriminators to improve the image quality. The left ventricle was contoured semiautomatically. Myocardial scar volume was quantified using the full width at half maximum method. Centerline chord method was used for scar transmurality measurement and visualized on bull's-eye plots. Linear regression, Pearson correlation (R), and intraclass correlation coefficients used for comparison of lesion quantification by VNE and LGE. Correspondingly, performed proof-of-principle histopathologic comparison of VNE in a porcine model of myocardial infarction.

Results: By five independent operators on 291 datasets on performing blinded analysis (all $p < 0.001$), VNE strongly correlated with LGE in quantifying scar size (R: 0.89; intraclass correlation coefficient: 0.94), and transmurality (R: 0.84; intraclass correlation coefficient: 0.90) in 66 patients (277 test datasets), and VNE provided significantly better image quality than LGE. Reviewed by two cardiovascular magnetic resonance experts all test image slices and noted an overall accuracy of 84% for VNE in detecting scars when compared with LGE, with specificity of 100% and sensitivity of 77%. With histopathology, an outstanding visuospatial agreement in two cases of a porcine model of myocardial infarction was presented by VNE.

Conclusion: For myocardial scar assessment in patients presented with earlier myocardial infarction, high agreement with LGE cardiovascular magnetic resonance in the visuospatial scattering and lesion quantification with higher image quality were revealed by VNE. A potentially transformative artificial intelligence-based technology (VNE) appears as an auspicious technique in decreasing time for scan and expenses, costs. In the near future, an increasing clinical throughput proved to be helpful in refining the accessibility of cardiovascular magnetic resonance.

ARTICLE COMMENTARY

Ischemic heart disease (IHD) is a global health concern, and late gadolinium enhancement (LGE) cardiac magnetic resonance (CMR) imaging is the standard for assessing myocardial scars and viability. While LGE-CMR provides accurate information, the use of contrast agents and lengthy scan times has led to the exploration of noninvasive, contrast-free techniques for more efficient and accessible CMR imaging in IHD management.

Native CMR methods, such as T1 mapping, offer contrast-free alternatives for cardiac phenotyping and detection of late gadolinium enhancement (LGE) abnormalities. Virtual native enhancement (VNE), an artificial intelligence (AI)-based approach, shows promise in generating LGE-like images from native T1 maps, providing a rapid and reliable assessment of myocardial scars and viability in patients with previous myocardial infarction. Further development of VNE holds potential for gadolinium-free visualization and quantification of myocardial scar burden with potential histopathologic validation.

A study conducted at the University of Oxford John Radcliffe Hospital used human CMR datasets from University of Oxford Center for Clinical Magnetic Resonance Research clinical service and the OxAMI study (Oxford Acute Myocardial Infarction quality assurance) to develop and validate the VNE technique. Quality assurance ensured matching slice positions, and a standardized phantom was used for T1 mapping quality control. The VNE generator, trained using U-Net streams, and conditional generative adversarial networks, fused cine frames, and T1 maps to produce contrast-free VNE images that resemble LGE images with improved clarity. Discriminators were trained to distinguish VNE and LGE images and assess image clarity. An additional convolutional layer was added to produce intermediate VNE signals that match LGE in pixelwise similarity, improving the interpretability of the deep learning process.

The VNE method was developed using data from 912 patients (4,271 datasets) with previous myocardial infarction. After quality control, 775 patients' data (3,002 datasets) were used for development, and 68 patients' data (291 datasets) were used for testing. Left ventricle contours were obtained semi-automatically, and scar volume and transmurality were quantified using specific methods. Quantification of lesions by VNE and LGE was compared using linear regression, Pearson correlation, and intraclass correlation coefficients. Additionally, a proof-of-principle histopathologic comparison of VNE was performed in a porcine model of myocardial infarction. Quantification of myocardial scars was performed on an independent test dataset of 277 VNE and conventional LGE images from 66 patients. In these patients, VNE demonstrated strong correlation with LGE in quantifying both infarct scar size and transmurality. There was high agreement in scar size (R = 0.89; ICC = 0.94) and scar transmurality (R = 0.84; ICC = 0.90), indicating the potential of VNE to replace LGE for noninvasive and contrast-free assessment of myocardial scars. There were no records of reported cases where VNE wrongly introduced a myocardial scar in LGE-negative slices. Generally, on CMR expert review metting, VNE revealed an accuracy of 84% in noticing a scar when compared with LGE, with a specificity of 100% and a sensitivity of 77%. VNE images generated from precontrast cine and native T1 maps were compared with LGE imaging and histopathology in a porcine test dataset ($n = 2$). VNE accurately depicted transmural myocardial infarction (MI) in the left anterior descending artery territory, with patterns, sizes, and extents of scars in high agreement with LGE. Quantitative infarct sizes showed good correlation between VNE and LGE. There was excellent agreement between VNE, LGE, macroscopic scarring on ex vivo slices, histologic evidence of infarction and fibrosis, and collagen accumulation on staining. This supports the reliability of VNE for noninvasive visualization and quantification of myocardial scars.

Virtual native enhancement technology, combining T1 mapping with cine imaging signals, improves sensitivity in detecting and quantifying myocardial scars compared to T1 mapping alone, as this may underestimate the extent and viability of infarction as T1 values of tissues in vivo can change over time, with chronic infarct scars developing lipomatous metaplasia and lower T1 values, while acute myocardial infarction can lead to overestimation of infarct size and transmurality on LGE due to myocardial edema and increased gadolinium contrast uptake. Implementing a robust quality control process is crucial for the clinical application of AI technologies, and incorporating an automated deep learning algorithm, manual inspection, and standardized image acquisition can enhance confidence in the reliability of generated images. Real-time image checking during scanning allows for confirmation of findings and ensuring sufficient image quality, potentially reducing the need for contrast administration. VNE technology offers superior image quality compared to LGE CMR, enables comprehensive myocardial scar assessment, and has the potential for quicker throughput in cardiac imaging protocols.

Further research is needed to expand VNE technology to cover a wider range of myocardial pathologies. Some patients' characteristics were not available in the retrospective data used for VNE development, and viability and prediction of functional recovery were not directly assessed in this study. Future development of VNE may enable the differentiation of acute pathologies beyond LGE, including edema-sensitive modalities like T2-based imaging.

ARTICLE 9

Validating an Idiopathic Dilated Cardiomyopathy Diagnosis using Cardiovascular Magnetic Resonance: The Dilated Cardiomyopathy Precision Medicine Study

Haas GJ, Zareba KM, Ni H, Bello-Pardo E, Huggins GS, Hershberger RE; Study Principal Investigator (PI) and Co-Investigators: The Ohio State University. Validating an Idiopathic Dilated Cardiomyopathy Diagnosis Using Cardiovascular Magnetic Resonance: The Dilated Cardiomyopathy Precision Medicine Study.
Circ Heart Fail. 2022;15(5):e008877.

Abstract

Background: Coronary artery disease (CAD) identified by coronary angiography has been essential to distinguish the etiology of dilated cardiomyopathy (DCM), including the assignment of idiopathic or ischemic cardiomyopathy. To identify myocardial scar and identify etiology, late gadolinium enhancement (LGE) with cardiovascular magnetic resonance (CMR) has appeared as an important approach.

Methods: Patients with left ventricular dilation and dysfunction attributed to idiopathic DCM were included in the DCM Precision Medicine Study. After, expert clinical review ischemic or other cardiomyopathies were excluded. CAD with >50% narrowing at angiography of ≥1 epicardial coronary artery has ischemic cardiomyopathy. For study inclusion, CMR was not required, but in a post-hoc analysis of available CMR reports, patterns of LGE were classified as no LGE, ischemic-pattern LGE—subendocardial/transmural, nonischemic LGE—midmyocardial/epicardial.

Results: A total of 1,204 idiopathic DCM patients were considered, out of which 396 (32.9%) had a prior CMR study; of these, 327 (82.6% of 396) had LGE imaging (mean age 46 years; 53.2% male; 55.4% white); 178 of the 327 (54.4%) exhibited LGE, and 156 of the 178 had LGE consistent with idiopathic DCM. The remaining 22 had transmural or subendocardial LGE. Of these 22, in 13 normal coronary angiography was observed, three showed luminal irregularities, one showed a distant thrombus, one has CAD with <50% coronary artery narrowing, data of four was not available.

Conclusion: In the DCM Precision Medicine Study, cohort who had LGE-CMR data is available of 327 enrolled probands. In 22 (6.7%), an ischemic-pattern of LGE was identified, all had idiopathic DCM as decided by expert clinical review.

ARTICLE COMMENTARY

The use of coronary angiography for identifying coronary artery disease (CAD) has been crucial in differentiating the causes of dilated cardiomyopathy (DCM), such as idiopathic or ischemic cardiomyopathy. However, cardiac magnetic resonance (CMR) with late gadolinium enhancement (LGE) has emerged as an alternative method for detecting myocardial scar and determining the etiology of DCM.

The Precision Medicine DCM Study is a multisite consortium aiming to investigate the genetic basis of idiopathic dilated cardiomyopathy (DCM) and assess the impact of a family communication intervention on clinical screening. The study planned to enroll 1,300 probands with idiopathic DCM and 2,600 of their relatives, with data analysis based on eligible probands who consented and were recruited by March 23, 2020. Diagnostic criteria include a left ventricular ejection fraction (LVEF) below 50% and left ventricular enlargement based on gender/height-specific thresholds. The study excluded patients with various conditions that could potentially cause nonidiopathic DCM.

A patient interview questionnaire collected demographic information, medical history, symptoms, past procedures and tests, genetic evaluations, lifestyle factors, and other relevant data. A structured medical record query form abstracted information on cardiovascular disease history, diagnostic testing, medication history, laboratory data, and primary and secondary diagnoses. The study database was used to identify patients who underwent comprehensive contrasted CMR examinations with LGE imaging, and their CMR reports were evaluated for specific parameters. The distributions of patients who had CMR imaging were compared to those without imaging. Statistical analyses were conducted to compare differences in percentages and means using appropriate tests such as Pearson Chi-square, Fisher's exact test (for small numbers), t-test, or ANOVA. A significance level of 0.05 was used. The presence of myocardial infarct scar identified by LGE was described in terms of counts and percentages of patients.

Among the 327 patients who underwent CMR with LGE imaging, 54.4% (178 patients) showed late gadolinium enhancement. Within this group, 6.7% (22 patients) exhibited LGE patterns associated with ischemic events, while 93.3% (156 patients) had nonischemic LGE patterns. Patients with ischemic-pattern LGE were older, had shorter duration of DCM, larger indexed LV volumes, and lower LVEF compared to those with nonischemic LGE. Among the 22 patients with ischemic-pattern LGE, 18 had available coronary angiographic data. Notably, three cases had luminal irregularities, one had moderate CAD, one had a coronary thrombus, and the remaining 13 had normal coronary angiography. Detailed evaluations of these cases provided additional insights into the etiology of their cardiomyopathy.

Cardiac magnetic resonance (CMR) with LGE imaging has been proposed as a valuable tool for determining the underlying causes of myocardial disease. LGE can identify fibrosis resulting from various factors, including prior myocardial infarction. In patients with DCM and no known CAD or prior myocardial infarction, LGE patterns can differentiate between ischemic and nonischemic etiologies. Patients with DCM having normal coronary angiography or minimal CAD point toward alternative mechanisms such as coronary artery embolus, repeated ischemic insults due to elevated wall stress, or genetic causes. The presence of ischemic-pattern LGE in idiopathic DCM can help with accurate phenotyping and potentially predict clinical outcomes. The study validated the clinical diagnostic criteria used in the DCM Precision Medicine Study and provided insights into LGE patterns in nonischemic DCM patients.

ARTICLE 10

Cardiac Magnetic Resonance Identifies Raised Left Ventricular Filling Pressure: Prognostic Implications

Garg P, Gosling R, Swoboda P, Jones R, Rothman A, Wild JM, et al. Cardiac magnetic resonance identifies raised left ventricular filling pressure: prognostic implications.
Eur Heart J. 2022;43(26):2511-22.

Abstract

Aims: In heart failure (HF), noninvasive imaging is routinely used to estimate left ventricular filling pressure (LVFP). For subphenotyping HF cardiovascular magnetic resonance (CMR) is emerging as an important imaging tool. Although, from CMR, presently LVFP cannot be estimated. This study aimed to inspect (i) in patients with suspected HF if CMR can estimate LVFP and (ii) if CMR-modeled LVFP has prognostic power.

Methods and results: All suspected HF patients go through right heart catheterization (RHC), CMR, and transthoracic echocardiography (TTE) (validation cohort only) within 24 hours of each other. RHC measured pulmonary capillary wedge pressure (PCWP) was used as a reference for LVFP. A total of 835 patients were enrolled (mean age: 65 + 13 years, 40% male). Death was considered as the primary endpoint at follow-up. Two CMR metrics were associated with RHC PCWP: LV mass and left-atrial volume in the derivation cohort ($n = 708$, 85%). When applied to the validation cohort ($n = 127$, 15%), the correlation coefficient between RHC, PCWP and CMR-modeled PCWP was 0.55 (95% CI 0.41–0.66, $p < 0.0001$). In classifying patients as normal or raised filling pressures (76% vs. 25%) CMR-modeled PCWP was superior to TTE. Found association of CMR-modeled PCWP with an increased risk of death (HR 1.77; $p < 0.001$). Kaplan–Meier analysis done to predict survival at 7-year follow-up (35% vs. 37%, $\chi^2 = 0.41$, $p = 0.52$), CMR-modeled PCWP was comparable to RHC PCWP ($\geq$15 mm Hg).

Conclusion: In patients with suspected HF a physiological CMR model can estimate LVFP. Additionally, CMR-modeled LVFP has a prognostic role.

ARTICLE COMMENTARY

Heart failure (HF) is a growing problem with significant social and economic implications. The main diagnostic method for HF is invasive catheter-based assessment of left ventricular filling pressure (LVFP). Noninvasive techniques like transthoracic echocardiography (TTE) are preferred, but lack precision. Cardiac magnetic resonance (CMR) imaging can provide detailed information and aid in HF diagnosis and sub-phenotyping. However, there is currently no CMR model available to predict LVFP or assess prognosis.

In a study conducted at a hospital in the UK by P Garg et al. over a period of 8 years, suspected heart failure (HF) patients underwent right heart catheterization (RHC), cardiac magnetic resonance (CMR), and transthoracic echocardiography (TTE) within 24 hours of each other. The pulmonary capillary wedge pressure (PCWP) measured by RHC was used as the reference for left ventricular filling pressure (LVFP). Death was considered the primary endpoint during follow-up. A total of 835 patients were enrolled with a mean age of 65 ± 13 years and 40% being male. In the derivation cohort ($n = 708$, 85%), two CMR measurements, LV mass, and left atrial volume were associated with RHC-measured PCWP and an equation was derived [CMR PCWP = 6.1352 + (0.07204 * LAV) + (0.02256 * LVM)]. When applied to the validation cohort ($n = 127$, 15%), the correlation coefficient between RHC PCWP and CMR-modeled PCWP was 0.55 (95% CI 0.41–0.66, $p < 0.0001$). CMR-modeled PCWP outperformed TTE in identifying patients with normal or raised filling pressures (76% vs. 25%). Kaplan–Meier analysis showed that CMR-modeled PCWP was comparable to RHC PCWP ($\geq$15 mm Hg) in predicting survival at the 7-year follow-up (35% vs. 37%). Both RHC-measured and CMR-modeled PCWP ($\geq$15 mm Hg) were comparable in predicting survival up to a maximum follow-up of 7 years. CMR-modeled PCWP showed a significant association with mortality even after adjusting for other CMR parameters.

The CMR model simplifies heart failure assessment by focusing on key parameters. Compared to invasive methods like RHC, CMR offers a noninvasive and cost-effective estimate of left ventricular filling pressure (LVFP). It demonstrates superior prognostic power and easy interpretation. However, it has limitations such as higher variability and a tendency to overestimate LVFP at higher values. This single-center observational study may have selection bias as it was conducted at a referral center for RHC assessment. The study included clinically stable, real-world patients with shortness of breath. The diagnostic accuracy of the CMR model for categorizing LVFP is good, but more research is needed for accurate quantification and risk stratification. Prospective studies are required to validate the proposed algorithm in a broader population. Comparison with TTE-based algorithms and advanced echocardiographic techniques was not performed in this study.

A physiological CMR model incorporating volumetric and functional metrics demonstrates accurate prediction of invasively measured PCWP and enhances classification compared to standard TTE models. Additionally, the prognostic value of CMR-modeled PCWP is comparable to RHC-measured PCWP.

REFERENCES

1. Harikrishnan S, Jeemon P, Ganapathi S, Agarwal A, Viswanathan S, Sreedharan M, et al. Five-year mortality and readmission rates in patients with heart failure in India: Results from the Trivandrum heart failure registry. Int J Card. 2021;326:139-43.
2. Ponikowski P, Voors AA, Anker SD, Bueno H, Cleland JG, Coats AJ, et al.; Authors/Task Force Members; Document Reviewers. 2016 ESC Guidelines for the diagnosis and treatment of acute and chronic heart failure: the task Force for the diagnosis and treatment of acute and chronic heart failure of the European Society of Cardiology (ESC).Developed with special contribution of the Heart Failure Association (HFA) of the ESC. Eur J Heart Fail. 2016;18:891-975.
3. Malagoli A, Rossi L, Zanni A, Sticozzi C, Piepoli MF, Benfari G. Quantified mitral regurgitation and left atrial function in heart failure with reduced ejection fraction: interplay and outcome implications. Eur J Heart Fail. 2022;24:694-702.
4. Inciardi RM, Pagnesi M, Lombardi CM, Anker SD, Cleland JG, Dickstein K, et al. Clinical implications of left atrial changes after optimization of medical therapy in patients with heart failure. Eur J Heart Fail. 2022;24:2131-9.
5. Benfari G, Antoine C, Essayagh B, Batista R, Maalouf J, Rossi A, et al. Functional mitral regurgitation outcome and grading in heart failure with reduced ejection fraction. JACC Cardiovasc Imaging. 2021;14:2303-15.

SECTION 4
Genetics in Heart Failure

Section Editor: Harikrishnan S

Co-Editors: Sudeep Kumar, Linda Koshy, Poonam Tripathi

ARTICLE 1

Risk Prognostication with Genotype versus Phenotype in Genetic Cardiomyopathies

Paldino A, Dal Ferro M, Stolfo D, Gandin I, Medo K, Graw S, et al. Risk Prognostication with Genotype vs Phenotype in Genetic Cardiomyopathies.
J Am Coll Cardiol. 2022;80(21):1981-94.

Abstract

Background: Phenotypic heterogeneity in cardiomyopathies (CMPs) occurred due to diverse genetic backgrounds. Previously genotype-phenotype correlation studies have mainly concentrated on singular phenotype platform. The different diagnostic and prognostic characteristics of the CMP genotype across different phenotypic expressions have not been explored in detail.

Objectives: The present study showed that the differences in outcome prediction were assessed by comparing genotype with phenotype at presentation in single large cohort comprising CMP and positive genetic testing.

Methods: The study enrolled 281 patients with 80% having dilated cardiomyopathy (DCM) along with other pathogenic or likely pathogenic variants including arrhythmogenic right ventricular cardiomyopathy, left-dominant arrhythmogenic cardiomyopathy (ACM), and biventricular ACM. The primary outcome comprised of all-cause death (D) or requirement for heart transplantation (HT) while secondary outcomes included sudden cardiac death (SCD) or major ventricular arrhythmias (MVA) and heart failure-related death (DHF) or HT or left ventricular assist device implantation (LVAD).

Results: Study showed that SCD and MVA events were more common often in those without DCM and in those with variants of *DSP*, *PKP2*, *LMNA*, and *FLNC* genes. The worst rates of D/HT and DHF/HT/LVAD were shown by LMNA.

The genotype-based classification was thus much better predictive of SCD/MVA after adjustment for age and sex compared to phenotype-based classification.

Conclusion: Heterogeneity is observed in genetic cardiomyopathies, genotypes were associated with significant phenotypic. However, in the present study, genotypic classification showed higher accuracy than phenotype classification in predicting the outcome of CMP patients. These findings support the risk stratification of patients with positive genetic testing, adding updated information to our current understanding of inherited CMPs.

ARTICLE COMMENTARY

Phenotype-only classification of cardiomyopathy (CMP) is what is followed in clinical settings, but it is challenging. The genetic background of the patient can significantly influence the prognostic stratification of CMPs. Palidino et al., 2023, in this study compared phenotypic versus genotypic CMP classification in predicting clinical outcomes. The phenotypes studied were in majority dilated cardiomyopathy (DCM) along with others like arrhythmogenic right ventricular cardiomyopathy (ARVC), arrhythmogenic left-dominant ventricular cardiomyopathy (ALVC), and biventricular (BiV) arrhythmogenic cardiomyopathy.

From 2016 to 2019, the study enrolled a total number of 834 patients affected by the DCM, ARVC, and others who were subjected to genetic testing. The pathogenic or likely pathogenic (P/LP) variants were around one-third of these. Their study endpoints were: (1) all-cause death (D) or heart transplantation (HT) as primary endpoint; (2) sudden cardiac death (SCD) or major ventricular arrhythmia (MVA) as arrhythmic secondary endpoint; and (3) heart failure-related death (DHF) or enlisting for HT or use of left ventricular assist device (LVAD) as HF secondary endpoint.

The follow-up of 118 months showed that genotypic classification better prognosticated the risk of SCD or MVA, and *LMNA* gene variants were having worse outcomes in terms of D/HT and DHF/HT/LVAD. This was particularly evident by how the phenotype at the onset would change after follow-up.

The application of a genotype-based classification in nonhypertrophic CMP cohort was found to be effective for identifying clinical characteristics relevant for future therapeutic management. For example, atrioventricular (AV) blocks and left bundle branch block (LBBB) in LMNA, atrial fibrillation (AF) in TTN and isolated RV dysfunction in *PKP2* were strongly corelated. The "arrhythmic genes" were identified as *LMNA, FLNC, DSP,* and *PKP2* and prompted further evaluation for implantable cardioverter-defibrillator implantation (ICD) irrespective of LV dysfunction. Therefore, they suggested that grouping cardiomyopathies with different causative gene provide a basis and understanding of disease-specific therapies. The authors identified the limitations of the study, as (1) magnetic resonance imaging data were not considered in their analysis. (2) There may have been unrecognized arrhythmic events that were experienced by patients but not captured by any phenotypic measures, leading to misclassification of some ACM into DCM. To summarize, genetic testing was found to supplement the process of defining the diagnosis for more accurate classification and management of nonhypertrophic CMPs and may be a step closer to precision medicine.

ARTICLE 2

Genotyping Indian Patients with Primary Cardiomyopathies-analysis of Database

Vaidya V, Dhiman RS, Mittal A, Khullar M, Sharma M, Bahl A. Genotyping Indian patients with Primary Cardiomyopathies-analysis of Database.
Indian Heart J. 2023;75(1):43-6.

Abstract

Introduction: There is a variation of genotype among each population. Limited data on genotyping on Indian cardiomyopathy patients is available.

Methods: Present study designed to analyze and generate a database of sequence variations in primary cardiomyopathies patients in Indian patients. All data of the cardiomyopathy cohort at the Postgraduate Institute of Medical Education and Research (PGIMER), Chandigarh was included. Furthermore, all published reports in PubMed using specific search terms were included, selected the only reports containing sequence variations in Indian cardiomyopathy patients till December 2020. Also, analyzed affected genes and sequence variations, methodologies, and quality of clinical data. Documented all the novel sequence variations.

Results: A record of 493 datasets including 417 different sequence variations was generated. From these datasets, 137 datasets are from the PGIMER database which consisting of 94 different variants. On considering Indian cardiomyopathy cohort from 2000 to 2020 only 63 publications were included for genotyping data with 335 sequence variations. Five (7.9%) studies were from institutions abroad. 35.1% variation were found to be novel from published variations. Selective genotyping was carried out by most studies. In only nine (14.3%) publications comprehensive genotyping using cardiomyopathy panels or whole exome sequencing was reported.

Conclusion: In Indian cardiomyopathy patients, database of 417 different sequence variations was analyzed. Here, we found novel sequence variation over a third of all reported sequence variations in Indians.

ARTICLE COMMENTARY

A comprehensive cardiomyopathy database of all sequence variations in the Indian population is crucial to understanding the degree of pathogenicity of rare variants and to assist in clinical decision making. In the paper published in the Indian Heart Journal in 2023, Vaidya et al. highlighted the paucity of genotyping data from Indian cardiomyopathy patients. They reported the creation of a database of sequence variations reported in Indian patients with primary cardiomyopathies, which included sequence variations in manuscripts published in PubMed indexed journals in a 20-year period from 2000 to 2020 along with unpublished data of a cardiomyopathy cohort at the Postgraduate Institute of Medical Education and Research (PGIMER), Chandigarh. Out of 3,623 publications during this period they found only 63 papers that included clinical studies, population-based studies, in silico, in vitro, and animal studies published on Indian patients.

A database of 493 datasets including 417 different sequence variations was created, of these, the PGIMER database had 137 datasets consisting of 94 different variants. It was interesting to note that the authors referred to "datasets" instead of absolute number of patients which implied that the same cohort of patients may have been repeatedly reused by research groups to screen different candidate genes using techniques such as "single-strand conformation polymorphism (SSCP)" and "Sanger sequencing". Therefore, their database was a collection of different variants reported by majority of papers that have employed candidate gene screening techniques and nine papers that used cardiomyopathy panels or whole exome sequencing. Following analysis, they reported summary counts of the number of publications in 5-year blocks, the genotyping methodologies used, the datasets available for different cardiomyopathies and the number of different variants in different genes. However, the specifics of the datasets or the gene variants were not reported.

The authors also discussed several limitations in the Indian data. This included sequencing of mutation hotspots, publication bias toward reporting of novel variants and sparce availability of clinical data of patients with rare variants. They mentioned that the choice of genes such as *MYH7*, *TNNT2*, and *MYBPC3* used for genotyping in HCM was driven by a priori hypotheses. Since cardiomyopathies are now known to be caused by ~3,000 pathogenic or likely pathogenic variants in as many as 107 genes, the candidate gene approach though economical has low genetic coverage, low throughput, and is subject to selection and publication bias. A classic example discussed was that of the 25-base pair (bp) deletion in intron-32 in the *MYBPC3* gene that is only found in individuals of South Asian descent. This is a common variant that has a minor allele frequency of 4% of the Indian population reportedly associated with hypertrophic cardiomyopathy, however, since its allele frequency transcends the actual disease frequency of 1 out of 500 (i.e., 0.2%), the observed association could be due to sampling bias. As per the American College of Medical Genetics and Genomics (ACMG), this variant is now classified as benign owing to the high prevalence in healthy population, having a higher prevalence than other clinically reported variants in the *MYBPC3* gene and being positioned in a nonconserved gene region. Moreover, the authors reckoned that incomplete reporting of clinical data, especially for rare variants, disallows conducting any analysis of association of variants with outcomes, assessment of its pathogenicity, and undermines the utility of genetic testing for cascade screening or in clinical decision-making. The authors concluded by pointing out an urgent need for a regularly updated comprehensive Indian database.

ARTICLE 3

Clinical Risk Score to Predict Pathogenic Genotypes in Patients with Dilated Cardiomyopathy

Escobar-Lopez L, Ochoa JP, Royuela A, Verdonschot JAJ, Dal Ferro M, Espinosa MA, et al. Clinical Risk Score to Predict Pathogenic Genotypes in Patients With Dilated Cardiomyopathy.
J Am Coll Cardiol. 2022;80(12):1115-26.

Abstract

Background: Genotyping in nonischemic dilated cardiomyopathy (NIDCM) or isolated left ventricular systolic dysfunction (LVSD) enables screening of family members and influences risk-stratification, but in a significant number of patients its result is negative, limiting its widespread acceptance for testing.

Objectives: This study aimed to externally validate and develop a score that predicted increased probability of a positive genetic test (G+) in dilated cardiomyopathy (DCM) or LVSD.

Methods: In a total of 1,015 genotyped patients from Spain with DCM/LVSD, clinical electrocardiogram and echocardiographic variables were collected. To identify variables independently predicting G+ multivariable logistic regression analysis was used which were summed to generate the Madrid Genotype Score. From the Maastricht and Trieste registries the external validation sample were comprised of 1,097 genotyped patients.

Results: A G+ result was found from the derivation and validation cohorts, 377 (37%) and 289 (26%) in patients respectively. The study revealed that a positive family history of DCM, clinically presence of skeletal myopathy and absence of hypertension along with low electrocardiogram QRS voltage and absence of left bundle branch block predicted probability of a positive genetic test. A score containing these factors predicted a G+ result, ranging from 3% when all predictors were absent to 79% when ≥4 predictors were present. By internal validation a C-statistic obtained of 0.74 (95% CI 0.71–0.77) and a calibration slope of 0.94 (95% CI 0.80–1.10). In the external validation cohort, the observed C-statistic was 0.74 (95% CI 0.71–0.78).

Conclusion: To predict a G+ result in DCM/LVSD, the Madrid Genotype Score is an accurate and reliable tool.

ARTICLE COMMENTARY

The developed Madrid Genotype Score emerged as a novel tool to predict positive genetic test results in nonischemic dilated cardiomyopathy (DCM)/left ventricular systolic dysfunction (LVSD). Escobar-Lopez et al., 2022, reported the construction of the Madrid Genotype Score for nonischemic dilated cardiomyopathy (NIDCM) or LVSD patients to predict pathogenic genotypes. They explained that although helpful, genetic testing is yet to develop as part of routine practice for work-up of DCM/LVSD. A relatively low detection rate and the perception that genetic findings have limited influence on patients' treatment were mentioned as challenges. Moreover, they cited that only 30–40% of DCM cases are caused by pathogenic or likely pathogenic (P/LP), with variants of unknown significance (VUS) found in >20% of cases. They opined that this would introduce more challenges to the clinician in variant interpretation and in communicating this information to patients and families. In this context, the Madrid Genotype Score was designed to predict a positive genetic test result in patients with DCM/LVSD, enabling identification of individuals with high probability of a positive genetic test.

In order to create the Madrid Genotype Score, they examined set of various parameters including 18 clinical variables, electrocardiogram characteristics, and echocardiographic variables in a cohort of DCM/LVSD patients from Spain. For external validation genotyped patients from the Maastricht and Trieste registries were assessed. Using multivariable logistic regression analysis, they identified five predictors to predict positive genetic test results namely positive family history for DCM, absence of hypertension or presence of skeletal muscle disease, absence of LBBB, and presence of low QRS voltage in peripheral electrocardiogram (ECG) leads. Their findings were congruent with previous reports demonstrating higher detection rates of P/LP variants in familial DCM; in cases manifesting skeletal myopathy which is considered a strong red flag due to the shared genetic etiology among some forms of genetic DCM and skeletal muscle disease; in low voltages on ECG which is described as a common finding in certain genotypes such as phospholamban (PLN) and desmosomal genes; and absence of left bundle branch block (LBBB) which is a potential role of desynchrony itself in LVSD.

The authors used a large sample size enabling testing of different spectrum of variables to develop the Madrid Genotype Score resulting in good levels of discrimination, that was subsequently validated in an independent external cohort. One limitation of the study was that not all patients underwent the same genetic analysis over different centers. Secondly, the derivation and validation cohorts were collected from inherited cardiac diseases units and tertiary DCM referral centers, respectively, limiting the application of the score to other cohorts of DCM with different characteristics.

Although at present, genetic testing is sparsely used in evaluation and work of DCM patients and family members screening, the authors in their expectation that genetic testing can become the routine practice in DCM/LVSD patients in near future have made their model available online as a "prediction calculator" with the following link, https://madriddcmscore.com.

ARTICLE 4

Genetic Architecture of Acute Myocarditis and the Overlap with Inherited Cardiomyopathy

Lota AS, Hazebroek MR, Theotokis P, Wassall R, Salmi S, Halliday BP, et al. Genetic Architecture of Acute Myocarditis and the Overlap with Inherited Cardiomyopathy.
Circulation. 2022;146(15):1123-34.

Abstract

Background: Acute myocarditis is an inflammatory condition that may function as a representative of the onset of dilated cardiomyopathy (DCM) or arrhythmogenic cardiomyopathy (ACM). In this present study, investigation of the frequency and clinical consequences of DCM and ACM genetic variants in a population-based cohort of patients with acute myocarditis was planned.

Material and methods: In this present study, authors inspected the frequency and clinical consequences of DCM and ACM genetic variants in a population-based cohort of patients with acute myocarditis. This was a population-based cohort of 336 consecutive patients with acute myocarditis enrolled in London and Maastricht. All participants underwent targeted DNA sequencing for well-characterized cardiomyopathy-associated genes with comparison to healthy controls ($n = 1,053$) sequenced on the same platform.

Results: Variants that would be considered pathogenic if found in a patient with DCM or ACM were identified in 8% of myocarditis cases compared with <1% of healthy controls ($p = 0.0097$). In the London cohort ($n = 230$; median age, 33 years; 84% men), patients were representative of national myocarditis admissions (median age, 32 years; 71% men; 66% case ascertainment), and there was enrichment of rare truncating variants (tvs) in ACM-associated genes [3.1% of cases vs. 0.4% of controls; odds ratio (OR) 8.2; $p = 0.001$]. In Maastricht ($n = 106$; median age: 54 years; 61% men), there was enrichment of rare tvs in DCM-associated genes, particularly TTN-tv, found in 7% [all with left ventricular ejection fraction (LVEF) < 50%] compared with 1% in controls (OR 3.6; $p = 0.0116$). There were no significant differences in family history between genotype-positive and genotype-negative cases in either London or Maastricht. There was a significant excess of truncating variants in *ACM* genes among cases compared with controls [3.0% vs. 0.4%; OR 8.2 (95% CI 2.4–28.4); $p < 0.001$], but no significant enrichment in *DCM* genes in aggregate or of TTN-tv.

Conclusion: We identified DCM- or ACM-associated genetic variants in 8% of patients with acute myocarditis. This was dominated by the identification of *DSP*-tv in those with normal LVFF and *TTN*-tv in those with reduced LVEF. Despite differences between cohorts, these variants have clinical implications for treatment, risk stratification, and family screening. Genetic counseling and testing should be considered in patients with acute myocarditis to help to reassure the majority while improving the management of those with an underlying genetic variant.

Although there were no significant differences in clinical outcomes by genotype status, our study was not powered to assess clinical outcomes, and the shorter follow-up in London may have contributed to the lower event rate in patients with ACM variants.

ARTICLE COMMENTARY

Acute myocarditis is an inflammatory condition that may function as the representative of the onset of dilated cardiomyopathy (DCM) or arrhythmogenic cardiomyopathy (ACM). Present study focuses on the important role of genetic sequencing in patients presenting with acute myocarditis and supports the concept that genotype-positive individuals may remain phenotypically silent until the occurrence of an environmental trigger. Here the author reports the first wide-ranging international genetic evaluation of patients with acute myocarditis to evaluate the frequency of genetic variants associated with inherited cardiomyopathies and, in particular, if truncating variants in TTN, a sarcomeric protein, are the most common in those genes which play an important role in development of left ventricular (LV) dysfunction. Authors hypothesized that myocarditis may act as an environmental modifier, initiating phenotypic expression of dilated cardiomyopathy (DCM) in previously healthy but genotype positive individuals attributable to an abnormal response to hemodynamic stress, as reported in other clinical settings. In contrast to London, there was a significant excess of truncating variants in *DCM* genes compared with controls [9.4% vs. 1.2%; odds ratio (OR) 7.4 (95% CI 3.1–17.8); $p < 0.001$], TTN-tv [6.6% vs. 0.9%; OR 8.2 (95% CI 3.0–22.5); $p < 0.001$], but no significant enrichment in *ACM* genes was observed. In present cohort, a total number of 1,230 cases with myocarditis were recruited from hospitals across Northwest London and evaluated by cardiovascular magnetic resonance (CMR) or immunohistopathology of myocardial tissue by the European Society of Cardiology criteria. Of which 114 were consecutively recruited <14 days after acute hospitalization, and 116 were retrospectively identified with CMR or biopsy-confirmed acute myocarditis. In Cohort 2, selected participants, i.e., 1,053 community-based healthy volunteers in London with no history of medical illness and no regular medication who were recruited through advertisements in the national media were considered. None were known to have had previous myocarditis. Normal cardiac structure and function were confirmed on noncontrast CMR. Variants that would be considered pathogenic if found in a patient with DCM or ACM were identified in 8% of myocarditis cases compared with <1% of healthy controls ($p = 0.0097$). In the London cohort ($n = 230$; median age, 33 years; 84% men), patients were representative of national myocarditis admissions, and there was enrichment of rare truncating variants in *ACM*-associated genes (3.1% of cases vs. 0.4% of controls; OR 8.2; $p = 0.001$). This was driven predominantly by DSP-tv in patients with normal left ventricular ejection fraction (LVEF) and ventricular arrhythmia. In Maastricht ($n = 106$; median age, 54 years; 61% men), there was enrichment of rare truncating variants in *DCM*-associated genes, TTN-tv, found in 7% compared with 1% in controls. Across both cohorts over a median of 5.0 years, all-cause mortality was 5.4%. Genetic evaluation identified pathogenic or likely pathogenic variants in cardiomyopathy-associated genes in 8% of patients presenting with acute myocarditis, demonstrating an overlap between myocarditis and inherited cardiomyopathy. The Northwest London cohort captured two-thirds of all adult admissions recorded in National Health Service (NHS) records within this population of 2.3 million. These patients were typically young, presenting with chest pain, troponin elevation, and a normal LVEF. The Maastricht cohort was older and more often had reduced LVEF and symptoms of heart failure. In this population, DCM variants were identified in 9.4% of cases, most commonly TTN-tv, with a trend toward higher mortality. Present study identified DCM- or ACM-associated genetic variants in 8% of patients with acute myocarditis. One in 13 cases with acute myocarditis harbored an underlying pathogenic or likely pathogenic variant in key cardiomyopathy-associated genes. This highlights the potential role of genetic sequencing in patients presenting with acute myocarditis and supports the concept that genotype-positive individuals may remain phenotypically silent until the occurrence of an environmental trigger. Further studies are required to dissect the mechanisms to help target therapy and to provide greater understanding of how genetic variants influence long-term clinical outcomes. However, sensitivity analyses confirmed that the key findings were not affected by ethnicity and remained significant when assessed against the 141,456 unrelated individuals in gnomAD. Third, although we selected genes that were robustly associated with cardiomyopathy, we did not include *FLNC*, which has recently gained interest as a result of involvement in the pathogenesis of left-dominant forms of ACM. Further studies are required to dissect the mechanisms to help target therapy and to provide greater understanding of how genetic variants influence long-term clinical outcomes. With the increasing prevalence of myocarditis secondary to immune checkpoint inhibitors and both coronavirus disease 2019 (COVID-19) infection and vaccination, our findings may provide understanding to guide susceptibility and risk stratification in these areas.

ARTICLE 5

The Response to Cardiac Resynchronization Therapy in LMNA Cardiomyopathy

Sidhu K, Castrini AI, Parikh V, Reza N, Owens A, Tremblay-Gravel M, et al. The response to cardiac resynchronization therapy in LMNA cardiomyopathy.
Eur J Heart Fail. 2022;24(4):685-93.

Abstract

Aims: Cardiac implantable electronic device (CIED) therapy is essential to the management of LMNA cardiomyopathy as atrioventricular block and ventricular tachyarrhythmias are common. Present study planned to explain the role of cardiac resynchronization therapy (CRT) in the effect of heart failure in LMNA cardiomyopathy.

Methods and results: Nine referral centers were initially recruited and retrospectively identified patients with *LMNA* cardiomyopathy undergoing CRT with available pre- and postechocardiograms. Factors associated with CRT response were acknowledged [defined as improvement in left ventricular ejection fraction (LVEF) ≥ 5% 6 months after-implant] and the associated impact on the primary outcome of death, implantation of a left ventricular assist device (LVAD) or cardiac transplantation was evaluated. Authors recognized 105 patients (mean age 51 ± 10 years) who were undergoing CRT, including 70 (67%) who underwent CRT as a CIED upgrade. The mean change in LVEF ~6 months post-CRT was +4 ± 9%. A CRT response occurred in 40 (38%) patients and was associated with lower baseline LVEF or a high percentage of right ventricular pacing prior to CRT in patients with preexisting CIED. In patients with a European Society of Cardiology class I guideline indication for CRT, response rates were 61%. The CRT response was evident at thresholds of LVEF ≤ 45% or percent pacing ≥50%. There was a 1.3-year estimated median difference in event-free survival in those who responded to CRT ($p = 0.04$).

> **Conclusion:** In short, present study concluded that in patients with LMNA cardiomyopathy who underwent CRT, an improvement in systolic function noted, particularly especially when the indications for implantation were strong. With limited options post-CRT progresses in LVEF are found to be associated with survival benefits in the current population.

ARTICLE COMMENTARY

Presence of dominant mutations in *LMNA* was reported approximately in 5% of patients who were presented with complaints of dilated cardiomyopathy and found to be linked with age-dependent penetrance of conduction disease and arrhythmia, are out of proportion to the severity of systolic dysfunction. Several recommendations suggested by numerous studies and recommended a selective criterion for implantable cardioverter defibrillator (ICD) implantation in *LMNA* cardiomyopathy patients with comparatively preserved systolic function. This study was planned to discover the response to cardiac resynchronization therapy (CRT) in *LMNA* cardiomyopathy focused on overall betterment in left ventricular systolic function. They assumed that patients presented with *LMNA* cardiomyopathy would satisfactorily respond to CRT due to their high rates of atrioventricular block and frequent right ventricular pacing from preexisting pacemakers and defibrillators. Here, authors inspected the link between a response to CRT and the development of end-stage HF which well thought-out as the primary composite of death, cardiac transplantation, or implantation of a left ventricular assist device (LVAD).

From the baseline the median time of the requested 6-month echo was 7.5 months. Excluded those patients who undertook LVAD implantation, cardiac transplantation, or died earlier to the 6-month of assessment. Echocardiographic indices including left ventricular ejection fraction (LVEF) and left ventricular end-diastolic dimension were recorded from evaluation of hospital information systems medical record.

For those patients who undertook CRT as an upgrade of prevailing device, a review of the cardiac implantable electronic device (CIED) interrogation prior to implantation for pre-CRT percentage of ventricular pacing considered. Post-CRT, device interrogation was used to get the percentage of biventricular pacing at 6 and 24 months. In both the left anterior oblique and right anterior oblique projections they studied CRT implantation reports for left ventricular lead position in the coronary sinus. Here, a defined CRT response and super-response as an increase in LVEF of 5% and 10%, respectively, after 6 months were selectively collected.

The baseline characteristics of the 105 patients who were found to be suitable for inclusion criteria of this study considered and stratified by knowing the 6-month response to CRT. In all patients, median follow-up time-period decided for post-CRT implantation was 3.5 years. In both the groups, clinical characteristics were typical of the *LMNA* cardiomyopathy referral population, with a high frequency of primary prevention ICDs and atrial arrhythmias.

Available echocardiographic data of 24 months in six patients post-CRT were used instead of unavailable 6-month data. They evaluated the determination of the appropriateness for CRT by following the guidelines of 2021 European Society of Cardiology on cardiac pacing and CRT.

Patients who have not meeting class I or IIa criteria were classified as having a nonclassic indication. At 6 and 24 months, other outcomes included mainly the change in LVEF and left ventricular end-diastolic diameter (LVEDD), the New York Heart Association (NYHA) class at 6 months and QRS duration post-CRT.

It was noted that 18 and 55 patients shown a class I or class IIa indication for CRT, respectively. The remaining 32 patients have not met the inclusion criteria or have not shown sufficient data with which to categorize the suggestion for CRT. The baseline characteristics which significantly differed between CRT responders and nonresponders were considered to be reduced LVEF and increased frequency of ventricular pacing prior to CRT. In a total of 41 patients, procedural documentation of left ventricular lead implantation was available.

However, complications occurred in 9% of patients and reported pocket hematoma, infection, and led dislodgment, and did not differ between responders and nonresponders.

A promising CRT response was observed to be maximum in patients presented with a class I indication for implantation compared to those with a class IIa indication, or without a classic indication for implantation. In the similar way, they inspected the frequency of CRT response among patients with a CIED prior to CRT upgrade at a threshold of pacing at 50%. Whether dichotomized at LVEF 45% or 35%, the patients with reduced LVEF had significantly greater possibility of CRT response of 44% and 50%, respectively; LVEF was noted to be stable in 17 patients; and LVEF found decreased by 5% in only nine patients.

In this present study, outcomes associated with the primary implantation or upgrades to CRT in patients with *LMNA* cardiomyopathy are explored. *LMNA* cardiomyopathy is a well-known disease in which single-chamber pacemakers and defibrillators are utilized previously in the course for heart block and ventricular tachyarrhythmias. Factors associated with a CRT response were shown a depressed LVEF pre-CRT and an increased percentage of pre-CRT ventricular pacing among patients who undertook CRT as an upgrade of an existing CIED. Depending on the selected criteria used upgrading in functional status can occur in up to 60–70% of patients. Only 13% of the *LMNA* cardiomyopathy patients presented here would have met the inclusion criteria for MADIT CRT and 29% would have met criteria for resynchronization-defibrillation for ambulatory heart failure trial investigators (RAFT), and despite this, found an improvement in mean LVEF at 6 months of 4 ± 9% with CRT. Furthermore, the response to CRT in patients who met these criteria was too high, i.e., ~70%. While the *LMNA* cardiomyopathy patients they present here shared some features typical of CRT responders, only a third had left bundle branch block (LBBB) and 74% were in atrial fibrillation (AF)/flutter typical representative of *LMNA*. Grounded on findings from the present study it was recommended that the absence of LBBB or the presence of AF applied to exclude consideration of CRT in *LMNA* heart disease.

SECTION 5

Drug Therapy in Heart Failure

Section Editor: AK Pancholia

Co-Editor: Akshaya Pradhan

ARTICLE 1

Dapagliflozin in Heart Failure with Mildly Reduced or Preserved Ejection Fraction: DELIVER Trial

Solomon SD, McMurray JJV, Claggett B, de Boer RA, DeMets D, Hernandez AF, et al. Dapagliflozin in heart failure with mildly reduced or preserved ejection fraction.
N Engl J Med. 2022;387(12):1089-98.

Abstract

Background: Among patients with chronic heart failure and a left ventricular ejection fraction, sodium-glucose cotransporter-2 (SGLT-2) inhibitors reduce the risk of hospitalization for heart failure and cardiovascular death of 40% or less. Limited is known about the effectiveness of SGLT-2 inhibitors in patients with a higher left ventricular ejection fraction.

Methods: In present study, 6,263 patients with heart failure and a left ventricular ejection fraction of >40% to receive dapagliflozin (at a dose of 10 mg once daily) or matching placebo were randomly assigned, along with usual therapy. Composite of worsening heart failure (which was defined as either an unplanned hospitalization for heart failure or an urgent visit for heart failure) or cardiovascular death is the primary outcome, as measured in a time-to-event analysis.

Results: The primary outcomes occurred in 512 of 3,131 patients (16.4%) in the dapagliflozin group and in 610 of 3,132 patients (19.5%) in the placebo group [hazard ratio 0.82; 95% confidence interval (CI) 0.73–0.92; $p < 0.001$], over an average time of 2.3 years. In the dapagliflozin group, worsening heart failure occurred in 368 patients (11.8%) and in 455 patients (14.5%) in the placebo group (hazard ratio 0.79; 95% CI 0.69–0.91); cardiovascular death occurred in 231 patients (7.4%) and 261 patients (8.3%), respectively (hazard ratio 0.88; 95% CI 0.74–1.05). In the dapagliflozin group, total events and symptom burden were lower than in the placebo group. Similar results were noted among patients with a left ventricular ejection fraction of 60% or more and those with a left ventricular ejection fraction of <60%, and in prespecified subgroups results were similar, including patients with or without diabetes. In the two groups, the incidence of adverse events was similar.

Conclusion: Combined risk of worsening heart failure or cardiovascular death among patients with heart failure and a mildly reduced or preserved ejection fraction is reduced by dapagliflozin.

ARTICLE COMMENTARY

Objective: The goal of the trial was to assess the safety and efficacy of dapagliflozin in patients with left ventricular ejection fraction (LVEF) >40%, irrespective of diabetes status.

Study design: Patients were randomized in a 1:1 fashion to either dapagliflozin 10 mg (n = 3,131) or matching placebo (n = 3,132). All the patients were receiving appropriate treatments for heart failure (HF).
- *Total screened*: 10,418
- *Total number of enrollees*: 6,263
- *Duration of follow-up*: 2.3 years (median)
- *Mean patient age*: 71.7 years
- *Percentage female*: 44%

Inclusion criteria:
- Age ≥40 years
- Evidence of structural heart disease
- Ejection fraction (EF) >40%
- Elevated B-type natriuretic peptide (BNP)

Other salient features/characteristics:
- Predominantly white (71%)
- *New York Heart Association (NYHA) functional class II*: 75%
- *Mean LVEF*: 54%
- *Type 2 diabetes mellitus (T2DM)*: 45%
- *Estimated glomerular filtration rate*: 61 mL/min/1.73 m^2

Result: The primary outcome, cardiovascular death, or worsening HF for dapagliflozin versus placebo was: 16.4% versus 19.5% [hazard ratio (HR) 0.82; 95% confidence interval (CI) 0.73–0.92, p < 0.001).
- *Cardiovascular death*: 7.4% versus 8.3% (HR 0.88; 95% CI 0.74–1.05)
- *HF hospitalization or urgent visit for HF*: 11.8% versus 14.5% (HR 0.79; 95% CI 0.69–0.91)

For the primary outcome, benefit was similar among patients with or without DM2, and for categories of baseline EF (≤49%, 50–59%, and ≥60%).

Secondary outcomes:
- *All-cause mortality*: 15.9% versus 16.8% (HR 0.94; 95% CI 0.83–1.0; p > 0.05)
- *Any amputation*: 0.6% versus 0.8%
- *Any major hypoglycemic event*: 0.2% versus 0.2%

Interpretation: The results of this trial indicate that dapagliflozin is superior to placebo in improving HF outcomes among patients with symptomatic stable mildly reduced or preserved LVEF (EF >40%), irrespective of diabetes status, duration of HF, and baseline NT-proBNP levels. Benefit is primarily driven by a reduction in HF hospitalizations, not mortality. The benefit of dapagliflozin was consistent across the range of frailty, baseline systolic blood pressure (SBP), and body mass index (BMI) categories studied.

Perspective: Similar to EMPEROR-Preserved, this trial also enrolled patients with near-normal or normal EFs, and shows a benefit in this patient population, irrespective of diabetes status. Compared to EMPEROR-Preserved, this trial showed no attenuation of benefit among patients with EF >60%.

Key messages

- Sodium-glucose cotransporte- 2 inhibitor (SGLT-2I), like dapagliflozin, is the first such molecule found to be effective in heart failure with preserved ejection fraction (HFpEF), where all other molecules which were effective in heart failure with reduced ejection fraction (HFrEF) have been failed in HFpEF.
- Taken in to the consideration of the results of DAPA-HF also the clinical benefits of dapagliflozin are robust across the spectrum of ejection fraction in chronic HF.
- Trial also addresses the benefit in patients with HFmrEF and HFimpEF, which was not been addressed in EMPEROR-PRESERVED.

ARTICLE 2

Combining Loop with Thiazide Diuretics for Decompensated Heart Failure: The CLOROTIC Trial

Trulls JC, Morales-Rull JL, Casado J, Carrera-Izquierdo M, Snchez-Marteles M, Conde-Martel A, et al. Combining loop with thiazide diuretics for decompensated heart failure: the CLOROTIC trial.
Eur Heart J. 2023;44(5):411-21.

Abstract

Aim: To evaluate whether the addition of hydrochlorothiazide (HCTZ) to intravenous furosemide is a safe and effective strategy for improving diuretic response in acute heart failure (AHF)

Methods and results: This is a prospective, double-blind, placebo-controlled trial, included patients with AHF randomized to receive HCTZ or placebo in addition to an intravenous furosemide regimen. Changes in bodyweight and patient-reported dyspnea 72 hours after randomization were the primary endpoints. Metrics of diuretic response and mortality/rehospitalizations at 30 and 90 days were the secondary outcomes. Also, they assessed safety outcomes (changes in renal function and/or electrolytes). 230 patients (48% women, 83 years) were randomized. Assigned patients to HCTZ at 72 hours were more likely to lose weight than those assigned to placebo [−2.3 vs. −1.5 kg; adjusted estimated difference (notionally 95% confidence interval) −1.14 (−1.84 to −0.42); $p = 0.002$], but no significant differences in patient-reported dyspnea were noted (area under the curve for visual analogue scale: 960 vs. 720; $p = 0.497$). After randomization, these results were similar in 96 hours. Greater 24 hours diuresis (1,775 vs. 1,400 mL; $p = 0.05$) and weight loss for each 40 mg of furosemide (at 72 and at 96 hours) ($p < 0.001$) shown by patients allocated to HCTZ. Impaired renal function shown by patients assigned to HCTZ (increase in creatinine > 26.5 μmol/L or decrease in eGFR >50%; 46.5 vs. 17.2%; $p < 0.001$), but between groups hyponatremia and hypokalemia were similar. In mortality or rehospitalizations, no differences were noted.

Conclusion: In patients with AHF, the addition of HCTZ to loop diuretic therapy improved diuretic response.

ARTICLE COMMENTARY

Objective: The goal of the trial was to compare changes in body weight and patient-reported dyspnea among patients with acute decompensated heart failure (HF) receiving intravenous (IV) loop diuretics with hydrochlorothiazide (HCTZ) versus placebo.

Study design: The CLOROTIC trial was a multicenter, randomized, double-blind, placebo-controlled trial of patients hospitalized with acute decompensated HF. Patients were randomized in 1:1 fashion to receive HCTZ ($n = 114$) or placebo ($n = 116$) for 5 days supplied as oral tablets. All patients were also on furosemide. Dose of HCTZ: estimated glomerular filtration rate (eGFR) >50 mL/min: 25 mg daily; 20–50 mL/min: 50 mg daily; and <20 mL/min: 100 mg daily. Uptitration or downtitration of study medication was not permitted, and its dose could only be adjusted based on changes in GFR during the treatment period. Patients could not be discharged during the 5-day randomized treatment period for close monitoring of adverse effects.

Inclusion criteria:
- Age >18 years
- Chronic heart failure (HF) (no criteria for etiology of HF or EF)
- Hospitalization within previous 24 hours for acute decompensated HF
- Treatment with oral loop diuretic ≥1 month prior to hospitalization
- IV furosemide dose between 80 mg and 240 mg daily

Exclusion criteria:
- Clinical instability (acute coronary syndrome, cardiogenic shock, or intensive care unit admission)
- Treatment with inotropic agents
- Treatment with any thiazide diuretic during the month before admission
- Requirement of renal replacement therapy
- Potassium ≤2.5 or sodium ≤125 at randomization

Other salient features/characteristics:
- New York Heart Association (NYHA) class III (51%) or NYHA class IV (10%)
- 60% with history of HF hospitalization in the previous 12 months
- *Median estimated glomerular filtration rate (eGFR)*: 43 mL/min/1.73 m^2
- *Median N-terminal pro-B-type natriuretic peptide (NT-proBNP)*: 4,672 pg/mL
- *Mean EF*: 55%; 65.3% of participants had EF >50%
- *Mean systolic blood pressure*: 125 mm Hg
- *Mean oral furosemide dose*: 80 mg/day

Principal findings: The coprimary outcome, adjusted changes in body weight from baseline to 72 hours of randomization, for HCTZ versus placebo, was −2.3 kg versus 1.5 kg ($p = 0.002$).

The co-primary outcome, change in patient-reported dyspnea from baseline to 72 hours of randomization using the visual analog scale, for HCTZ versus placebo, was mean area under the curve (AUC) at 72 hours: 960 versus 720 ($p = 0.50$).

Key secondary outcomes for HCTZ versus placebo:
- *Change in weight at 96 hours*: −2.5 kg versus 1.5 kg ($p < 0.001$)
- *24-hour diuresis quantification*: 1,775 mL versus 1,400 mL ($p = 0.05$)
- *Hospital length of stay*: 7.0 versus 7.0 ($p = 0.17$)
- *All-cause mortality at 30 days*: 9.6% versus 6.0% ($p = 0.44$)
- *All-cause rehospitalization at 30 days*: 23.7% versus 16.4% ($p = 0.22$)
- *Impaired renal function*: 46.5% versus 17.2% ($p < 0.001$)

- *Increase in creatinine >26.5 µmol/L*: 46.5% versus 17.2% ($p < 0.001$)
- *Potassium levels ≤3.5 mmoL/L*: 44.7% versus 19.0% ($p < 0.001$)

Interpretation: Adding HCTZ to the IV loop diuretic enhances its diuretic effect with no change in patient-reported dyspnea. There is weight reduction at both 72 and 96 hours in HCTZ arm compared to those receiving placebo therapy. Though there are increases in hypokalemia, creatinine, and impaired renal function with HCTZ but differences in all-cause mortality or all-cause rehospitalization at 30 and 90 days.

Key messages

- In patients hospitalized for acute decompensated heart failure (ADHF), complete or residual congestion is commonly seen with loop diuretics.
- A substantial benefit in the congestion is seen when thiazide diuretics are added to loop diuretics with greater reduction of weight and VAS dyspnea scale in patients hospitalized with ADHF.
- There is a need of long-term safety trials using thiazide in these patients.

ARTICLE 3

Acetazolamide in Decompensated Heart Failure with Volume Overload: The ADVOR Trial

Mullens W, Dauw J, Martens P, Verbrugge FH, Nijst P, Meekers E, et al. Acetazolamide in acute decompensated heart failure with volume overload: The ADVOR Trial.
N Engl J Med. 2022;387(13):1185-95.

Abstract

Background: Till date, it is unclear whether acetazolamide, a carbonic anhydrase inhibitor that reduces proximal tubular sodium reabsorption, can improve the efficiency of loop diuretics, potentially leading to more and faster decongestion in patients with acute decompensated heart failure with volume overload.

Methods: This is a multicenter, parallel-group, double-blind, randomized, placebo-controlled trial, where enrolled those patients who were presented with acute decompensated heart failure, clinical signs of volume overload (i.e., edema, pleural effusion, or ascites), and an N-terminal pro–B-type natriuretic peptide (NT-proBNP) level of >1,000 pg/mL or a B-type natriuretic peptide level of >250 pg/mL to receive either intravenous acetazolamide (500 mg once daily) or placebo added to standardized intravenous loop diuretics (at a dose equivalent to twice the oral maintenance dose). According to the left ventricular ejection fraction (≤40% or >40%), randomization was stratified. The primary endpoint was composite of successful decongestion, defined as the absence of signs of volume overload, within 3 days after randomization and without an indication for escalation of decongestive therapy. The secondary endpoints of the study are a composite of death from any cause or rehospitalization for heart failure during 3 months of follow-up and safety was also considered.

Results: A total of 519 patients go through randomization and successful decongestion occurred only in the acetazolamide group in 108 of 256 patients (42.2%) and in the placebo group 79 of 259 (30.5%) [risk ratio 1.46; 95% confidence interval (CI) 1.17–1.82; $p < 0.001$]. Death from any cause or rehospitalization for heart failure happened in 76 of 256 patients (29.7%) in the acetazolamide group and in 72 of 259 patients (27.8%) in the placebo group (hazard ratio 1.07; 95% CI 0.78–1.48). Acetazolamide treatment was associated with higher cumulative urine output and natriuresis, findings consistent with better diuretic efficiency. In the two groups, the incidence of worsening kidney function, hypokalemia, hypotension, and adverse events was similar.

Conclusion: The addition of acetazolamide to loop diuretic therapy in patients with acute decompensated heart failure resulted in a greater incidence of successful decongestion.

ARTICLE COMMENTARY

Objective: The goal of the trial was to compare incidence of successful decongestion among patients with acute decompensated heart failure receiving intravenous (IV) loop diuretics with IV acetazolamide versus placebo.

Study design: The ADVOR trial was a multicenter, randomized, parallel group, double-blind, placebo-controlled trial of patients hospitalized with acute decompensated heart failure. Patient were randomized in 1:1 fashion to IV bolus of acetazolamide (500 mg daily, n = 259) or matching placebo (n = 260). Oral loop diuretics were given intravenously at double the oral maintenance dose over split doses. Participants received acetazolamide or placebo simultaneously with first dose of loop diuretics each day.

Inclusion criteria:
- Clinical signs of volume overload (edema, pleural effusion, and ascites)
- N-terminal pro–B-type natriuretic peptide (NT-proBNP) >1000 pg/mL or BNP >250 pg/mL
- Oral maintenance therapy with 40 mg of furosemide, 20 mg of torsemide, 1 mg of bumetanide, or more for ≥1 month prior to randomization

Exclusion criteria:
- Receipt of acetazolamide maintenance therapy
- Treatment with a sodium-glucose cotransporter-2 inhibitor (SGLT-2I)
- Systolic blood pressure <90 mm Hg
- Estimated glomerular filtration rate <20 mL/min/1.73 m^2
- Treatment with dose >80 mg IV furosemide equivalent during index hospitalization

Result: The primary outcome, successful decongestion within 3 days after randomization, for acetazolamide versus placebo, was: 42.2% vs. 30.5% ($p < 0.001$).

Key secondary outcomes for IV acetazolamide versus placebo:
- *Duration of hospital stay*: 8.8 days versus 9.9 days ($p = 0.016$)
- *All-cause mortality or rehospitalization for heart failure during 3-month follow-up*:

29.7% versus 27.8% (not statistically significant)
- *Combined renal safety endpoint*: 2.7% versus 0.8% ($p = 0.10$)
- *Hypokalemia*: 5.5% versus 3.9% ($p = 0.39$); hypotension: 6.6% versus 3.5% ($p = 0.11$)

Effect across baseline left ventricular ejection fraction: Acetazolamide resulted in improved diuretic response measured by higher cumulative diuresis and natriuresis and shortened length of stay without treatment effect modification by baseline left ventricular ejection fraction (LVEF) and it has been observed in all EF groups (>0.05).

Interpretation: Results suggest that irrespective of the baseline EF, adding IV acetazolamide to the loop diuretic in acute decompensated heart failure (ADHF) led to significantly greater incidence of successful decongestion within 3 days of randomization as compared with placebo. The study is limited in that it was exclusively performed in Belgium, which may limit generalizability across other racial/ethnic groups.

Key messages
- Achieving successful decongestion is a big challenge among patients with acute decompensated heart failure.
- Patients with residual congestion have a higher risk of post-discharge adverse outcomes.
- The current study provides strong evidence to support use of IV acetazolamide to achieve decongestion among patients with decompensated heart failure.
- Availability of IV acetazolamide is another challenge in India.

ARTICLE 4

Effects of Empagliflozin on Symptoms, Physical Limitations, and Quality of Life in Patients Hospitalized for Acute Heart Failure: Results from the EMPULSE Trial

Kosiborod MN, Angermann CE, Collins SP, Teerlink JR, Ponikowski P, Biegus J, et al. Effects of empagliflozin on symptoms, physical limitations, and quality of life in patients hospitalized for acute heart failure: Results from the EMPULSE trial. *Circulation. 2022;146(4):279-88.*

Abstract

Background: Poor health status, including a high burden of symptoms and physical limitations, and poor quality of life were experienced by patients hospitalized for acute heart failure. In chronic heart failure, sodium-glucose cotransporter-2 inhibitors (SGLT-2Is) improve health status, but their effect on these outcomes in acute heart failure is not well understood. Here, in this present study, investigation of the effects of the SGLT-2I empagliflozin on symptoms, physical limitations, and quality of life, using the Kansas City Cardiomyopathy Questionnaire (KCCQ) in the EMPULSE trial (Empagliflozin in Patients Hospitalized With Acute Heart Failure Who Have Been Stabilized) were planned.

Methods: Patients hospitalized for about 90 days, for acute heart failure were randomized to empagliflozin 10 mg daily or placebo. The KCCQ was evaluated at randomization and 15, 30, and 90 days. Examined the post hoc across the tertiles of baseline KCCQ-TSS for the effects of empagliflozin on the primary end point of clinical benefit [hierarchical composite of all-cause death, heart failure events, and a 5-point or greater difference in KCCQ total symptom score (TSS) change from baseline to 90 days]. Changes (randomization to day 90) in KCCQ domains, including TSS, physical limitations, quality of life, clinical summary and overall summary scores were evaluated in prespecified analyses using a repeated measures model.

Results: A total of 530 patients were randomized (265 each arm). Overall, baseline KCCQ-TSS was low [mean (SD), 40.8 (24.0) points]. Across the range of KCCQ-TSS, empagliflozin-treated patients experienced greater clinical benefit, with no treatment effect heterogeneity {win ratio [95% confidence intervals (CIs)] from lowest to highest tertile: 1.49 (1.01–2.20), 1.37 (0.94–1.99), and 1.48 (1.00–2.20) respectively; $p\ value$ for interaction=0.94}. Observed beneficial effects of empagliflozin on health status as early as 15 days and persisted through 90 days, at which point empagliflozin-treated patients experienced a greater improvement in KCCQ-TSS, physical limitations, quality of life, clinical summary, and overall summary [placebo-adjusted mean differences (95% CI) 4.45 (95% CI 0.32–8.59), $p = 0.03$; 4.80 (95% CI 0.00–9.61), $p = 0.05$; 4.66 (95% CI 0.32–9.01), $p = 0.04$; 4.85 (95% CI 0.77–8.92), $p = 0.02$; and 4.40 points (95% CI 0.33–8.48), $p = 0.03$, respectively].

Conclusion: In hospitalized patients, initiation of empagliflozin for acute heart failure produces clinical benefit irrespective of the degree of symptomatic impairment at baseline, and improved symptoms, physical limitations, and quality of life, with benefits seen as early as 15 days and maintained through 90 days.

ARTICLE COMMENTARY

Objective: The goal of the trial was to evaluate empagliflozin compared with placebo among patients with acute decompensated heart failure. Empagliflozin has been shown to reduce the risk of cardiovascular death or heart failure hospitalization among patients with chronic heart failure.

Study design:
- Randomized
- Parallel

Method: Participants with acute heart failure were randomized to empagliflozin 10 mg daily ($n = 265$) versus placebo ($n = 265$).
- *Total number of enrollees*: 530
- *Duration of follow-up*: 90 days
- *Mean patient age*: 71 years
- *Percentage female*: 33%
- *Percentage with diabetes*: 47%

Inclusion criteria:
- Patients admitted to the hospital with acute heart failure regardless of ejection fraction or diabetes status
- Systolic blood pressure ≥100 mm Hg and no symptoms of hypotension within 6 hours
- No increase in intravenous (IV) diuretic dose within 6 hours
- No IV vasodilators, including nitrates, within 6 hours
- No IV inotropic drugs within 24 hours

- N-terminal pro–B-type natriuretic peptide (NT-proBNP) ≥1,600 pg/mL or BNP ≥400 pg/mL during hospitalization or within 72 hours prior to admission

Other salient features/characteristics:
- *Median left ventricular ejection fraction*: 31%

Result:
Primary outcomes: The primary analysis was assessed by a stratified win ratio, defined as a composite of death, number of heart failure events, time to first heart failure event, and change in Kansas City Cardiomyopathy Questionnaire–Total Symptom Score (KCCQ-TSS) from baseline to 90 days. Clinical benefit occurred at a rate of 53.9% in the empagliflozin group compared with 39.7% in the placebo group ($p = 0.0054$).

Secondary outcomes:
- *Death*: 4.2% in the empagliflozin group versus 8.3% in the placebo group
- *Heart failure event*: 10.6% in the empagliflozin group versus 14.7% in the placebo group
- *Change in KCCQ-TSS*: 4.5 points for the empagliflozin group versus the placebo group ($p = 0.035$)
- *Acute renal failure*: 7.7% in the empagliflozin group versus 12.1% in the placebo group
- *Body weight change*: –1.5 kg for the empagliflozin group versus the placebo group ($p = 0.014$)

Effects of empagliflozin on quality of life: Patients were divided into tertiles based on Kansas City Cardiomyopathy Questionnaire-Total Symptom Score (KCCQ-TSS) (comparisons for empagliflozin versus placebo; p for interaction = 0.94).
- *Low tertile*: Win ratio, 1.49
- *Middle tertile*: Win ratio, 1.37
- *High tertile*: Win ratio, 1.48

Effects of empagliflozin on weight loss:
- Body weight change (kg) from baseline to day 15: –3.20 kg in the empagliflozin group versus –1.23 in the placebo group ($p < 0.0001$)
- Body weight change (kg) from baseline to day 30: –3.19 kg in the empagliflozin group versus –1.45 in the placebo group ($p = 0.0007$)
- Body weight change (kg) from baseline to day 90: –2.36 kg in the empagliflozin group versus –0.83 in the placebo group ($p = 0.014$)

Interpretation: This trial was extended to see the benefit of SGLT-2I in patients with acute decompensated heart failure (ADHF). Results are encouraging as we see a significant clinical benefit at 90 days compared with placebo with fewer deaths, reduction in body weight (decongestion), and improvement in the quality of life (QOL) in the empagliflozin arm. The results observed are regardless of ejection fraction or diabetes status.

Key messages
- The 1st month following hospitalization for heart failure is a particularly vulnerable time for patients.
- Targeting this vulnerable period is very important to prevent further hospitalizations or death which has been observed in this study with empagliflozin.

ARTICLE 5

Torsemide Comparison with Furosemide for Management of Heart Failure: TRANSFORM-HF Trial

Mentz RJ, Anstrom KJ, Eisenstein EL, Sapp S, Greene SJ, Morgan S, et al. Effect of Torsemide vs Furosemide After Discharge on All-Cause Mortality in Patients Hospitalized With Heart Failure: The TRANSFORM-HF Randomized Clinical Trial.
JAMA. 2023;329(3):214-23.

Abstract

Importance: In patients with heart failure, furosemide is consistently used loop diuretic, although several studies advocated a potential benefit for torsemide.

Objective: Present study is designed to determine whether torsemide results in decreased mortality on comparison with furosemide among hospitalized heart failure patients.

Design, setting, and participants: TRANSFORM-HF was an open-label, pragmatic randomized trial. In this trial, a total of 2,859 participants recruited who were hospitalized with heart failure condition (regardless of ejection fraction) at 60 hospitals in the United States. From June 2018 to March 2022, patients were recruited, with follow-up of 30 months for death and for hospitalizations 12 months. July 2022 was the final date for follow-up data collection.

Interventions: Investigator selected the dosage for loop diuretic strategy of torsemide (*n* = 1,431) or furosemide (*n* = 1,428).

Main outcomes and measures: All-cause mortality was primary outcome in analysis of time-to-event. All-cause mortality or all-cause hospitalization and total hospitalizations were 5 secondary outcomes assessed over 12 months, being highest in the hierarchy. Torsemide would reduce all-cause mortality by 20% compared with furosemide was the pre-specified primary hypothesis.

Results: A total of 2,859 participants with a median age of 65 years (IQR 56–75), 36.9% were women and 33.9% were Black in randomized TRANSFORM-HF trail. A total of 113 patients [53 (3.7%) in the torsemide group and 60 (4.2%) in the furosemide group] were withdrew consent from the trial prior to completion over a median follow-up of 17.4 months. In the torsemide group, death occurred in 373 of 1,431 patients (26.1%) and in the furosemide group 374 of 1,428 patients (26.2%) {hazard ratio 1.02 [95% confidence interval (CI) 0.89–1.18]}. All-cause mortality or all-cause hospitalization observed in 677 patients (47.3%) in the torsemide group and 704 patients (49.3%) in the furosemide group [hazard ratio 0.92 (95% CI 0.83–1.02)] over 12 months following randomization. Among 536 participants in the torsemide group, there were 940 total hospitalizations and among 577 participants in the furosemide group, 987 total hospitalizations [rate ratio 0.94 (95% CI 0.84–1.07)]. Similar results were observed in prespecified subgroups, including among patients with reduced, mildly reduced, or preserved ejection fraction.

Conclusion and relevance: Torsemide compared with furosemide did not result in a significant difference in all-cause mortality over 12 months among patients discharged after hospitalization for heart failure. Though, exact description of the findings obtained from this study is limited because of loss to follow-up, participant crossover, and nonadherence.

ARTICLE COMMENTARY

Objective: To determine whether torsemide results in decreased mortality compared with furosemide among patients hospitalized for heart failure.

Design, setting, and participants: TRANSFORM-HF was an open-label, pragmatic randomized trial that recruited 2,859 participants hospitalized with heart failure (regardless of ejection fraction) at 60 hospitals in the United States. Recruitment occurred from June 2018 through March 2022, with follow-up through 30 months for death and 12 months for hospitalizations.

Inclusion criteria:
- Patient hospitalized (≥24 hours) with worsening of chronic HF, or new diagnosis of heart failure and meets one of the following criteria:
  - A left ventricular ejection fraction (EF) ≤40% within 24 months prior to and including index hospitalization by any method
  - An elevated natriuretic peptide level (either NT-pro-B-type natriuretic peptide or B-type natriuretic peptide) during index hospitalization
- Plan for a daily outpatient oral loop diuretic regimen upon hospital discharge with anticipated need for long-term loop diuretic use
- ≥18 years
- Signed informed consent

Exclusion criteria:
- End-stage renal disease requiring renal replacement therapy
- Inability or unwillingness to comply with study requirements
- Implanted left ventricular assist device or implant anticipated <3 months
- Pregnant or nursing women
- Malignancy or other noncardiac condition limiting life expectancy to <12 months
- Known hypersensitivity to furosemide, torsemide, or related agents

Interventions: Loop diuretic strategy of torsemide ($n = 1,431$) or furosemide ($n = 1,428$) with investigator-selected dosage.

Main outcomes and measures: The primary outcome was all-cause mortality in a time-to-event analysis. There were five secondary outcomes with all-cause mortality or all-cause hospitalization and total hospitalizations assessed over 12 months being highest in the hierarchy. The prespecified primary hypothesis was that torsemide would reduce all-cause mortality by 20% compared with furosemide.

Results: Death occurred in 373 of 1,431 patients (26.1%) in the torsemide group and 374 of 1,428 patients (26.2%) in the furosemide group [hazard ratio 1.02 (95% CI 0.89–1.18)]. Over 12 months following randomization, all-cause mortality or all-cause hospitalization occurred in 677 patients (47.3%) in the torsemide group and 704 patients (49.3%) in the furosemide group [hazard ratio 0.92 (95% CI 0.83–1.02)]. There were 940 total hospitalizations among 536 participants in the torsemide group and 987 total hospitalizations among 577 participants in the furosemide group [rate ratio 0.94 (95% CI 0.84–1.07)]. Results were similar across prespecified subgroups, including among patients with reduced, mildly reduced, or preserved ejection fraction.

Conclusion and relevance: There is no significant difference in all cause mortality over 1 year between torsemide and furosemide in patients who are discharged after hospitalization for HF.

Key messages

- The long-standing question, whether frusemide is better or torsemide is better in patients hospitalized for heart failure, has been answered in this trial.
- No big difference between these medications has been observed in hospitalized patients for HF.
- This data cannot be extrapolated in patients treated outside the hospital.

ARTICLE 6

Virtual Care Team-guided Strategy Optimizes GDMT for Hospitalized HF Patients: The IMPLEMENT-HF Trial

Bhatt AS, Varshney AS, Moscone A, Claggett BL, Miao ZM, Chatur S, et al. Virtual Care Team-Guided Strategy Optimizes GDMT for Hospitalized HF Patients: The IMPLEMENT-HF Trial.
J Am Coll Cardiol. 2023;81(17):1680-93.

Abstract

Background: Optimization of the guideline-directed medical therapy (GDMT) to figure out scalable and safe approaches for heart failure.

Objectives: Present study planned to assess the safety and effectiveness of a virtual care team-guided strategy on GDMT optimization in hospitalized heart failure patients with reduced ejection fraction (HFrEF).

Methods: This is a multicenter implementation trial. A total of 252 hospital enrolled patients with left ventricular ejection fraction ≤40% to a virtual care team-guided strategy (107 encounters among 83 patients) or usual care (145 encounters among 115 patients) across 3 centers allocated in an integrated health system. In the team of virtual care group, clinicians received up to 1 daily GDMT optimization suggestion from a physician-pharmacist team. The primary outcome of the study was in-hospital change in GDMT optimization score (+2 initiations, +1 dose up-titrations, −1 dose down-titrations, −2 discontinuations summed across classes). By an independent clinical events committee, hospital safety outcomes were settled.

Results: The mean age was 69 ±14 years, among a total encounters of 252, out of which 85 (34%) were women, 35 (14%) were Black, and 43 (17%) were Hispanic. It was observed that the virtual care team strategy significantly showed improved GDMT optimization scores versus usual care (adjusted difference +1.2; 95% CI 0.7–1.8; $p < 0.001$). During hospitalization, new initiations (44% vs. 23%; absolute difference +21%; $p = 0.001$) and net intensifications (44% vs. 24%; absolute difference +20%; $p = 0.002$) were higher in the virtual care team group, translating to a number needed to intervene of 5 encounters. Generally, 23 (21%) in the virtual care team group and 40 (28%) in usual care experienced one or more adverse events ($p = 0.30$). Between groups, acute kidney injury, bradycardia, hypotension, hyperkalemia, and hospital length of stay were mostly similar.

Conclusion: In patients who hospitalized with HFrEF, it was observed that a virtual care team-guided strategy for GDMT optimization was safe. In an integrated health system also, an improved GDMT was reported across multiple hospitals. To optimize GDMT, virtual teams represent a centralized and scalable approach.

ARTICLE COMMENTARY

Aim: Implementation of guideline-directed medical therapy (GDMT) for heart failure with reduced ejection fraction (HFrEF) remains incomplete. Noncardiovascular hospitalization may present opportunities for GDMT optimization. Trial assessed the efficacy and durability of a virtual, multidisciplinary "GDMT team" on medical therapy prescription for HFrEF.

Methods: This study has allocated patients with a left ventricular ejection fraction (LVEF) ≤40% to a virtual care team-guided strategy (107 encounters among 83 patients) or usual care (145 encounters among 115 patients). The patients were from three centers in an integrated health care delivery system. Their mean age was 69 years, 34% were women, 14% were Black, and 17% were Hispanic.

Clinicians in the virtual care team group received up to once daily recommendations for optimizing GDMT from a physician-pharmacist team. The primary goal was to improve early treatment of four major drugs classes [beta-blockers; angiotensin-converting enzyme inhibitors (ACEIs)/ angiotensin receptor blocker (ARB)/ angiotensin receptor neprilysin inhibitor (ARNI); mineralocorticoid receptor antagonists; and sodium-glucose cotransporter-2 inhibitors (SGLT-2Is)].Effectiveness was measured by the in-hospital change in the optimization score (+2 initiations, +1 dose uptitrations, –1 downtitrations, –2 discontinuations summed across classes), and in-hospital safety outcomes were analyzed by an independent clinical events committee.

Results: Results showed that GDMT optimization scores improved with the virtual care team strategy versus usual care (adjusted difference +1.2; 95% CI 0.7–1.8; $p < 0.001$). In these groups respectively, there was a higher rate of new initiation of GDMT (44% vs. 23%; $p = 0.001$) and intensifications of ≥1 GDMT (50% vs. 28%; $p = 0.001$). This translated to a number-needed-to-intervene of five encounters to optimize GDMT during hospitalization.

In terms of safety outcomes, there was no significant excess in adjudicated serious adverse events (21% vs. 28%) in the intervention and control groups, respectively, had one or more safety events ($p = 0.30$), with similar rates of acute kidney injury, bradycardia, hypotension, and hyperkalemia.

Key messages
- This strategy represents a potential highly effective, scalable intervention that can lead to accelerated implementation of guideline concordant heart failure with reduced ejection fraction (HFrEF) care.
- This implementation strategy warrants testing in a large, multicenter, prospective, and randomized clinical trial.

ARTICLE 7

Effect of Sacubitril/Valsartan versus Valsartan on Left Atrial Volume in Patients with Pre-heart Failure with Preserved Ejection Fraction: The PARABLE Randomized Clinical Trial

Ledwidge M, Dodd JD, Ryan F, Sweeney C, McDonald K, Fox R, et al. Effect of Sacubitril/Valsartan vs Valsartan on Left Atrial Volume in Patients with Pre-Heart Failure with Preserved Ejection Fraction: The PARABLE Randomized Clinical Trial. *JAMA Cardiol. 2023;8(4):366-75.*

Abstract

Importance: A common condition pre-heart failure with preserved ejection fraction (pre-HFpEF) has no specific therapy apart from cardiovascular risk factor management.

Objective: To investigate the hypothesis that sacubitril/valsartan vs valsartan would reduce left atrial volume index using volumetric cardiac magnetic resonance imaging in patients with pre-HFpEF.

Design, setting, and participants: In Patients with Natriuretic Peptide Elevation (PARABLE) trial, the personalized prospective comparison of ARNI (angiotensin receptor/neprilysin inhibitor) with ARB (angiotensin-receptor blocker) was done. It was a prospective, double-blind, double-dummy, randomized clinical trial conducted over 18 months from April 2015 to June 2021. In Dublin, Ireland present study was carried out at single outpatient cardiology center. Out of 1,460 patients in the STOP-HF program or outpatient cardiology clinics, 461 were found to be perfect for initial criteria and were selected for inclusion in the study. 323 were further screened and 250 were found to be asymptomatic patients of 40 years and older with hypertension or diabetes, with elevated B-type natriuretic peptide (BNP) >20 pg/mL or N-terminal pro-B-type natriuretic peptide (NT-proBNP) >100 pg/mL, and were included patients with left atrial volume index >28 mL/m^2, and preserved ejection fraction observed to be >50%.

Results: Present study was designed to investigate the hypothesis that sacubitril/valsartan versus valsartan plays important role for reducing left atrial volume index by using volumetric cardiac magnetic resonance imaging in pre-HFpEF patients.

Interventions: Patients were randomized to angiotensin receptor neprilysin inhibitor sacubitril/valsartan titrated to 200 mg twice daily or matching angiotensin receptor blocker valsartan titrated to 160 mg twice daily.

Main outcomes and measures: Maximal left atrial volume index and left ventricular end diastolic volume index, ambulatory pulse pressure, NT-proBNP, and adverse cardiovascular events.

Results: Among the total 250 participants for this study, the median (IQR) age was considered 72.0 (68.0–77.0) years. In this study, they enrolled 154 men participants (61.6%) and 96 (38.4%) women. Most of patients [n = 245 (98.0%)] had hypertension and 60 (24.0%) had type 2 diabetes mellitus. In both groups, maximal left atrial volume index was increased in patients assigned to receive sacubitril/valsartan [6.9 mL/m^2; 95% confidence interval (CI) 0.0–13.7] versus valsartan (0.7 mL/m^2; 95% CI −6.3 to 7.7; $p < 0.001$) despite reduced markers of filling pressure. In the sacubitril/valsartan group, changes in pulse pressure and N-terminal pro-BNP were observed to be lower (−4.2 mm Hg; 95% CI −7.2 to −1.21 and −17.7%; 95% CI −36.9 to 7.4, respectively; $p < 0.001$) compared to the valsartan group (−1.2 mm Hg; 95% CI −4.1 to 1.7 and 9.4%; 95% CI −15.6 to 4.9, respectively; $p < 0.001$). In six patients (4.9%), major adverse cardiovascular events happened who are assigned to sacubitril/valsartan and 17 patients were (13.3%) assigned to receive valsartan (adjusted hazard ratio 0.38; 95% CI 0.17–0.89; adjusted $p = 0.04$).

Conclusion and relevance: Sacubitril/valsartan treatment was observed to be associated with a greater increase in left atrial volume index and improved markers of cardiovascular risk compared to valsartan, in current trial of patients with pre-HFpEF. Further research work is currently needed to better understand the observed increased cardiac volumes and long-term effects of sacubitril/valsartan in pre-HFpEF patients.

ARTICLE COMMENTARY

Objective: To investigate the hypothesis that sacubitril/valsartan versus valsartan would reduce left atrial volume index using volumetric cardiac magnetic resonance imaging in patients with pre-HFpEF.

Design, setting, and participants: The Personalized Prospective Comparison of ARNI (angiotensin receptor/neprilysin inhibitor) with ARB (angiotensin receptor blocker) in PARABLE (Patients with Natriuretic Peptide Elevation) trial was a prospective, double-blind, double-dummy, randomized clinical trial carried out over 18 months between April 2015 and June 2021. The study was conducted at a single outpatient cardiology center in Dublin, Ireland. Of 1,460 patients in the STOP-HF program or outpatient cardiology clinics, 461 met initial criteria and were approached for inclusion. Of these, 323 were screened and 250 asymptomatic patients 40 years and older with hypertension or diabetes, elevated B-type natriuretic peptide (BNP) > 20 pg/mL or N-terminal pro-B-type natriuretic peptide >100 pg/mL, left atrial volume index (NT-proBNP) >28 mL/m^2, and preserved ejection fraction >50% were included.

Interventions: Patients were randomized to ARNI sacubitril/valsartan titrated to 200 mg twice daily or matching angiotensin receptor blocker valsartan titrated to 160 mg twice daily.

Main outcomes and measures: Maximal left atrial volume index and left ventricular end diastolic volume index, ambulatory pulse pressure, NT-proBNP, and adverse cardiovascular events.

Results: Among the 250 participants in this study, the median (IQR) age was 72.0 (68.0–77.0) years; 154 participants (61.6%) were men and 96 (38.4%) were women. Most [$n = 245$ (98.0%)] had hypertension and 60 (24.0%) had type 2 diabetes mellitus. Maximal left atrial volume index was increased in patients assigned to receive sacubitril/valsartan (6.9 mL/m^2; 95% CI 0.0–13.7) versus valsartan (0.7 mL/m^2; 95% CI −6.3 to 7.7; $p < 0.001$) despite reduced markers of filling pressure in both groups. Changes in pulse pressure and NT-proBNP were lower in the sacubitril/valsartan group (−4.2 mm Hg; 95% CI, −7.2 to −1.21 and −17.7%; 95% CI −36.9 to 7.4, respectively; $p < 0.001$) than the valsartan group (−1.2 mm Hg; 95% CI −4.1 to 1.7 and 9.4%; 95% CI −15.6 to 4.9, respectively;

$p < 0.001$). Major adverse cardiovascular events occurred in six patients (4.9%) assigned to sacubitril/valsartan and 17 (13.3%) assigned to receive valsartan (adjusted hazard ratio 0.38; 95% CI 0.17–0.89; adjusted $p = 0.04$).

Conclusion and relevance: Sacubitril/valsartan showed a greater increase in left atrial volume index and improved markers of cardiovascular risk compared to valsartan in pre-heart failure with preserved ejection fraction (HFpEF) patients.

Key message

- Identification of pre-heart failure (stage B HF) is important because it is associated with increased HF and cardiovascular risk. It has been endorsed in the 2022 American Heart Association (AHA)/American College of Cardiology (ACC) guidelines for management of HF also. These patients should be targeted in the early stage of HF to prevent them to progress to further stage.

ARTICLE 8

Effect of Omecamtiv Mecarbil on Exercise Capacity in Chronic Heart Failure with Reduced Ejection Fraction: The METEORIC-HF Randomized Clinical Trial

Lewis GD, Voors AA, Cohen-Solal A, Metra M, Whellan DJ, Ezekowitz JA, et al. Effect of Omecamtiv Mecarbil on Exercise Capacity in Chronic Heart Failure With Reduced Ejection Fraction: The METEORIC-HF Randomized Clinical Trial. JAMA. 2022;328(3):259-69.

Abstract

Importance: Cardinal manifestation of heart failure with reduced ejection fraction (HFrEF) is mainly exercise limitation but is not steadily improved by any of the currently available guideline-directed medical therapies.

Objective: Present study was designed to determine whether omecamtiv mecarbil is a novel direct myosin activator that improves cardiac performance and responsible for reduction in the risk for cardiovascular death or first HF event in HFrEF and can improve peak exercise capacity in patients presented with chronic HFrEF.

Design, setting, and participants: This is a phase 3, double-blind, placebo-controlled randomized trial of HFrEF patients (left ventricular ejection fraction 35%) presented with New York Heart Association class II-III symptoms, N-terminal pro-B-type natriuretic peptide (NT-proBNP) level was found to be of 200 pg/mL or greater, and baseline peak oxygen uptake (VO$_2$) of 75% or less predicted was predicated. From March 2019 to May 2021, patients were randomized in a 2:1 ratio (omecamtiv mecarbil to placebo) at 63 sites in North America and Europe, with the record of last patient visit on November 29, 2021.

Interventions: Given orally twice daily at a dose of 25 mg, 37.5 mg, or 50 mg based on target plasma levels, omecamtiv mecarbil ($n = 185$) or matching placebo ($n = 91$), for about 20 weeks.

Main outcomes and measures: The primary end point of the study was a variation in exercise capacity (peak VO_2) from baseline to week 20. Total workload, ventilatory efficiency, and daily physical activity as determined by accelerometry were the secondary end points of the study.

Results: Among 276 selected and randomized patients [median age, 64 years; IQR, 55–70 years; only 42 women (15%)], 249 (90%) completed the trial. The considered median left ventricular ejection fraction was 28% (IQR 21–33) and the median baseline peak VO_2 was 14.2 mL/kg/min (IQR 11.6–17.4) in the omecamtiv mecarbil group and in the placebo group 15.0 mL/kg/min (IQR 12.0–17.2). Mean change in peak VO_2 did not differ significantly between the omecamtiv mecarbil and placebo groups [mean, −0.24 mL/kg/min vs. 0.21 mL/kg/min; least square mean difference, −0.45 mL/kg/min (95% CI −1.02 to 0.13); $p = 0.13$]. Dizziness (omecamtiv mecarbil: 4.9%, placebo: 5.5%), fatigue (omecamtiv mecarbil: 4.9%, placebo: 4.4%), heart failure events (omecamtiv mecarbil: 4.9%, placebo: 4.4%), death (omecamtiv mecarbil: 1.6%, placebo: 1.1%), stroke (omecamtiv mecarbil: 0.5%, placebo: 1.1%), and myocardial infarction (omecamtiv mecarbil: 0%, placebo: 1.1%) are the adverse events.

Conclusion and relevance: Omecamtiv mecarbil over 20 weeks did not significantly improve exercise capacity compared with placebo in patients with chronic HFrEF. For improvement of exercise capacity, findings of present study do not support the use of omecamtiv mecarbil for treatment of HFrEF patients.

ARTICLE COMMENTARY

Objective: To determine whether omecamtiv mecarbil, a novel direct myosin activator that improves cardiac performance and reduces the risk for cardiovascular death or first heart failure (HF) event in heart failure with reduced ejection fraction (HFrEF), can improve peak exercise capacity in patients with chronic HFrEF.

Design, setting, and participants: This is a Phase 3, double-blind, placebo-controlled randomized trial of patients with HFrEF (left ventricular ejection fraction ≤35%), in NYHA class II-III symptoms. N-terminal pro-B-type natriuretic peptide (NT-proBNP) level of 200 pg/mL or greater, and baseline peak oxygen uptake (VO_2) of 75% or less of predicted. Patients were randomized in a 2:1 ratio (omecamtiv mecarbil to placebo) between March 2019 and May 2021 at 63 sites in North America and Europe.

Interventions: Omecamtiv mecarbil ($n = 185$) or matching placebo ($n = 91$), given orally twice daily at a dose of 25 mg, 37.5 mg, or 50 mg based on target plasma levels, for 20 weeks.

Outcome measures: The primary end point was a change in exercise capacity (peak VO_2) from baseline to week 20. Secondary end points included total workload, ventilatory efficiency, and daily physical activity as determined by accelerometry.

Results: Among 276 patients who were randomized [median age, 64 years; IQR 55–70 years; 42 women (15%)], 249 (90%) completed the trial. The median left ventricular ejection fraction was 28% (IQR

21-33) and the median baseline peak VO$_2$ was 14.2 mL/kg/min (IQR 11.6-17.4) in the omecamtiv mecarbil group and 15.0 mL/kg/min (IQR 12.0-17.2) in the placebo group. Mean change in peak VO$_2$ did not differ significantly between the omecamtiv mecarbil and placebo groups {mean, –0.24 mL/kg/min vs. 0.21 mL/kg/min; least square mean difference, –0.45 mL/kg/min [95% confidence interval (CI) –1.02 to 0.13]; $p = 0.13$}. Adverse events included dizziness (omecamtiv mecarbil: 4.9%, placebo: 5.5%), fatigue (omecamtiv mecarbil: 4.9%, placebo: 4.4%), heart failure events (omecamtiv mecarbil: 4.9%, placebo: 4.4%), death (omecamtiv mecarbil: 1.6%, placebo: 1.1%), stroke (omecamtiv mecarbil: 0.5%, placebo: 1.1%), and myocardial infarction (omecamtiv mecarbil: 0%, placebo: 1.1%).

Conclusion and relevance: No significant improvement has been observed with omecamtiv mecarbil in patients with chronic HFrEF compared with placebo regarding exercise capacity over 20 weeks. These findings do not support the use of omecamtiv mecarbil in this scenario.

Key messages
- Improvement in quality of life (QOL) is an important area in any pharmacotherapy trial in CVD.
- Previous trial with omecamtiv mecarbil in HFrEF (GALACTIC-HF) showed a lower incidence of a composite of a heart failure event or death from cardiovascular causes.
- But in this trial, a paradox has been observed where omecamtiv mecarbil has shown no improvement in exercise capacity. This is not the first study where:
  - Medication that improves outcomes in one trial but does not improve exercise capacity in another trial in same population.

ARTICLE 9

Study of Dietary Sodium Intervention Under 100 mmol in Heart Failure (SODIUM-HF): An International, Open-label, Randomized, Controlled Trial

Ezekowitz JA, Colin-Ramirez E, Ross H, Escobedo J, Macdonald P, Troughton R, et al. SODIUM-HF Investigators. Study of Dietary Sodium Intervention Under 100 mmol in Heart Failure (SODIUM-HF): An International, Open-Label, Randomized, Controlled Trial.
Lancet. 2022;399(10333):1391-400.

Abstract
Background: Patients with heart failure have shown that dietary restriction of sodium may help to prevent fluid overload and adverse outcomes. So, present study was designed to investigate dietary intervention under 100 mmol in heart failure patients (SODIUM-HF). This study was planned to test whether or not a reduction in dietary sodium helpful in the reduction of the incidence of future clinical events.

Methods: In this study, patients were enrolled at 26 sites in six countries (Australia, Canada, Chile, Colombia, Mexico, and New Zealand). It is an international, open-label, randomized, and controlled trial (SODIUM-HF). Patients with chronic heart failure [New York Heart Association (NYHA) functional class II–III] and were aged 18 years or older also getting optimally tolerated guideline-directed medical treatment. Using a standard number generator, patients were randomly given (1:1) and varying block sizes of two, four, or six, stratified by site, to either usual care according to local guidelines or a low sodium diet of < 100 mmol (i.e., <1,500 mg/day). The composite of cardiovascular-related admission to hospital, departmental visit for cardiovascular-related emergency, or all-cause death within 12 months in the intention-to-treat (ITT) population (i.e., all randomly assigned patients) is the primary outcome of the study. They have assessed safety in the current ITT population.

Findings: A total of 806 patients were randomly given to a low sodium diet ($n = 397$) or usual care ($n = 409$) from March 24, 2014 to December 9, 2020. Median age was 67 years (IQR 58–74) and for women 268 (33%) and for men 538 (66%). The median sodium intake decreased from 2,286 mg/day (IQR 1,653–3,005) to 1,658 mg/day (1,301–2,189) in the low sodium group between baseline and 12 months and in the usual care group from 2,119 mg/day (1,673–2,804) to 2,073 mg/day (1,541-2,900). In the low-sodium diet group, events comprising the primary outcome had occurred in 60 (15%) of 397 patients and 70 (17%) of 409 in the usual care group {hazard ratio (HR) 0.89 [95% confidence interval (CI) 0.63–1.26; $p = 0.53$] by 12 months. In 22 (6%) all-cause death occurred in patients of the low-sodium diet group and 17 (4%) in the usual care group [HR 1.38 (0.73–2.60); $p = 0.32$], in 40 (10%) cardiovascular-related hospitalization noted in patients of the low-sodium diet group and 51 (12%) patients in the usual care group [HR 0.82 (0.54–1.24); $p = 0.36$], and noted departmental visits in 17 (4%) patients in the low-sodium diet group cardiovascular-related emergency and in the usual care group 15 (4%) patients [HR 1.21 (0.60–2.41); $p = 0.60$]. Not observed any safety events related to the study treatment in either of the group.

Interpretation: A dietary intervention to reduce sodium intake did not reduce clinical events in ambulatory patients with heart failure.

ARTICLE COMMENTARY

Objective: The goal of the trial was to evaluate a low-sodium diet compared with usual care among ambulatory patients with heart failure.

Study design:
- Randomized
- Parallel
- Open-label
- Stratified

Patients with New York Heart Association (NYHA) class II–III heart failure symptoms on optimal medical therapy were randomized to a low-sodium diet (<1,500 mg daily) ($n = 397$) versus usual care ($n = 409$).
- *Total number of enrollees*: 806
- *Duration of follow-up*: 12 months
- *Mean patient age*: 66 years
- *Percentage female*: 32%
- *Percentage with diabetes*: 33%

Inclusion criteria:
- Patients ≥18 years of age with heart failure (preserved or reduced left ventricular systolic function)

- NYHA class II–III symptoms
- End-stage renal disease on hemodialysis
- Uncontrolled thyroid or end-stage liver failure
- Cardiac device or revascularization in the previous month or planned in the next 3 months
- Hospitalization for cardiovascular cause in the last month
- Uncontrolled atrial fibrillation
- Active malignancy with expected lifespan <2 years
- Poor compliance with the study protocol
- Enrollment in another study

Exclusion criteria:
- Average daily sodium intake <1,500 mg
- Serum sodium <130 mmol/L

Other salient features/characteristics:
- *Mean ejection fraction*: 36%
- *Atrial fibrillation*: 39%
- At 12 months, dietary sodium intake was 1,658 mg in the low-sodium diet group versus 2,073 mg in the usual care group ($p < 0.0001$).

Result: The trial was terminated early due to impact from the coronavirus disease 2019 (COVID-19) pandemic.

Primary outcome:
- All-cause mortality, or cardiovascular emergency department visit/hospitalization at 12 months, occurred in 15% of the low-sodium group versus 17% of the usual care group [hazard ratio (HR) 0.89; $p = 0.53$].

Secondary outcomes:
- *All-cause mortality at 12 months*: 6% of the low-sodium group versus 4% of the usual care group (HR 1.38; $p = 0.32$)
- The difference in the adjusted mean Kansas City Cardiomyopathy Questionnaire (KCCQ) overall summary score at 12 months was 3.38 points greater in the low-sodium group versus usual care group ($p = 0.011$).
- The difference in the adjusted mean 6-minute walk test at 12 months was 6.6 minutes greater in the low-sodium group versus usual care group ($p = 0.41$).

Interpretation: There is no reduction in adverse cardiovascular (CV) events with low-sodium diet in ambulatory patients with heart failure although there is a modest improvement in quality of life; unfortunately, interpretation of the findings was limited as trial was terminated early.

Key messages
- Trial is super exciting and really transforms the way we counsel patients about sodium restriction.
- Trial result is going to change our advisory statement what we tell to our patients about salt removing strict from restriction.

ARTICLE 10

Electronic Alerts to Improve Heart Failure Therapy in Outpatient Practice: A Cluster Randomized Trial

Ghazi L, Yamamoto Y, Riello RJ, Coronel-Moreno C, Martin M, O'Connor KD, Simonov M, et al. Electronic alerts to improve heart failure therapy in outpatient practice: A Cluster Randomized Trial.
J Am Coll Cardiol. 2022;79(22):2203-13.

Abstract

Background: Present study aimed to examine whether targeted and tailored electronic health record (EHR) alerts recommending GDMT in eligible HFrEF (heart failure with reduced ejection fraction) patients improve GDMT use.

Methods: A realistic, EHR-based, cluster-randomized comparative effectiveness trial was PROMPT-HF (PRagmatic trial Of Messaging to Providers about Treatment of Heart Failure). A total of 100 providers caring for HFrEF patients were randomized to either an alert or usual care. Along with patient characteristics, the alert notified providers of individual GDMT recommendations. Increase in the number of GDMT classes prescribed at 30 days post-randomization was primary outcome for this study. Here, providers' knowledge about guidelines and user experience were surveyed.

Results: In present study, 1,310 ambulatory patients with HFrEF were enrolled from April to October 2021. Participants' median age was 72 years, comprises 31% female, 18% Black, and 32% median left ventricular ejection fraction. B-blockers were received by 84% of participants, 71% received a renin–angiotensin–aldosterone system inhibitor, 29% received a mineralocorticoid receptor antagonist, and 11% received a sodium-glucose cotransporter-2 inhibitor, at baseline. Out of 685, only 176 (26%) participants in the alert arm versus 117 of 625 (19%) in the usual care arm, thus GDMT class prescription increasing by >40% after alert exposure [adjusted relative risk 1.41; 95% confidence interval (CI) 1.03–1.93; $p = 0.03$]; these are the major primary outcome. The number of patients needed to alert to result in an increase in addition of GDMT classes was 14. The alert was effective at enabling improved prescription of medical therapy for HF agreed by a total of 79% of alerted providers.

Conclusion: For outpatients with HFrEF, led to significant higher rates of GDMT at 30 days when equated with usual care, here used a real-time, targeted, and tailored EHR-based alerting system for analysis. In heart failures, this low-cost intervention can be rapidly assimilated into clinical care and may accelerate adoption of high-value therapies.

ARTICLE COMMENTARY

Objective: Do targeted and tailored electronic health record (EHR) alerts recommending guideline-directed medical therapy (GDMT) for patients with heart failure with reduced ejection fraction (HFrEF) improve medication use?

Methods: The PROMPT-HF is a pragmatic, single health-system, EHR-based, cluster-randomized (by provider), comparative effectiveness trial. Retrospectively, the top 100 providers caring for HFrEF patients in the outpatient setting (physicians or advanced practice providers) were identified. These providers were randomized to receive a best practice alert (BPA) for patients with HFrEF or no alert at the time of an outpatient visit. Patients were enrolled from April, 2021 to October, 2021.

Inclusion criteria: For patients included age ≥18 years, left ventricular ejection fraction (LVEF) ≤40%, and not already on all four classes of GDMT for HFrEF [beta-blockers (BBs), renin–angiotensin–aldosterone system (RAAS) inhibitors, mineralocorticoid receptor antagonists (MRAs), sodium-glucose cotransporter-2 inhibitors (SGLT-2Is)].

Exclusion criteria: For patients included those who have opted out of EHR-based research and in hospice care. In addition, providers completed a pre- and post-study survey assessing knowledge and comfort levels. The post-study survey also assessed user experience with the BPA.

Alert information:
- BPA triggered when opening order entry module.
- *Information provided*: Current LVEF, blood pressure, heart rate, serum potassium and creatinine levels, estimated glomerular filtration rate.
- *Recommendations provided*: All four classes of medication displayed. Medication classes missing were highlighted and allergies were noted. Links to an order set with missing medications and indications were provided.

The primary outcome was proportion of patients with an increase in the number of GDMT classes prescribed at 30 days. The secondary outcomes were increase in dose of currently prescribed GDMT, filling of prescriptions, total healthcare costs, hospitalizations, emergency department visits, and death.

Results: There were 1,310 ambulatory patients with HFrEF enrolled, who were managed by the 100 providers randomized. The providers consisted of 69% physicians and 31% advanced practice providers. Patient characteristics were well balanced between the intervention and control groups. At baseline, among all the patients, 84% were on a BB, 71% were on a RAAS inhibitor, 29% were on an MRA, and 11% were on an SGLT-2I.

Primary outcome: 25.7% of patients had an increase in the number of GDMT classes at 30 days in the alert arm compared to 18.7% in the no alert arm [adjusted relative risk 1.41; 95% confidence interval (CI) 1.03–1.93; $p = 0.03$]. The number needed to treat/alert was 14. Broken down by class for alert compared to no alert, increases were seen in 5.8 versus 2.9% for BBs ($p = 0.007$), 7.7% versus 7.0% for RAAS inhibitors ($p = 0.22$), 7.6% versus 5.3% for MRAs ($p = 0.20$), and 9.8% versus 7.5% for SGLT-2I ($p = 0.41$).

Conclusion: Targeted and tailored EHR BPAs for outpatient HFrEF visits led to significantly higher rates of GDMT initiation at 30 days compared with usual care (no BPAs).

Key message

- There is a need for a better outcome in HFrEF patients by proper optimization of GDMT by healthcare providers (HCP) and systems. Results of this study is promising in order to overcome clinical inertia by HCP.

ARTICLE 11

Safety, Tolerability, and Efficacy of Up-titration of Guideline-directed Medical Therapies for Acute Heart Failure (STRONG-HF): A Multinational, Open-label, Randomized Trial

Mebazaa A, Davison B, Chioncel O, Cohen-Solal A, Diaz R, Filippatos G, et al. Safety, tolerability and efficacy of up-titration of guideline-directed medical therapies for acute heart failure (STRONG-HF): a multinational, open-label, randomised, trial.
Lancet. 2022;400(10367):1938-52.

Abstract

Aim: Acute heart failure (HF) patients are at high risk of readmission to hospital and death, particularly in the 90 days following discharge time. Present study aimed to assess the safety and efficacy of early optimization of oral HF therapy with beta-blockers (BB), angiotensin-converting enzyme inhibitors (ACEIs) or angiotensin receptor blockers (ARBs) or angiotensin receptor–neprilysin inhibitors (ARNIs), and mineralocorticoid receptor antagonists (MRA) on 90-day clinical outcomes in patients admitted for acute HF.

Methods: It is a multicenter, randomized, open-label, parallel-group study. A total of 900 patients were enrolled and randomized in a 1:1 ratio to either "usual care" or "high-intensity care". Patients selected for the study in usual care arm will be discharged and at the site managed according to usual clinical practice. Before discharge in the high-intensity care arm, doses of oral HF medications—including a BB, ACEI or ARB, and MRA—uptitrated to 50% of recommended doses and to 100% of recommended doses within 2 weeks of discharge. If the patients develop worsening symptoms, uptitration will be delayed and signs of congestion, hyperkalemia, hypotension, bradycardia, worsening of renal function, or significant increase in N-terminal pro-B-type natriuretic peptide (NT-proBNP) levels were observed between visits. The primary endpoint of the study was 90-day all-cause mortality or HF readmission.

Conclusion: This STRONG-HF is the first reported study to assess whether rapid uptitration of evidence-based guideline-recommended therapies with close follow-up in a large cohort of patients discharged from an acute HF admission is safe and during the first 90 days after discharge can it affect adverse outcomes.

ARTICLE COMMENTARY

Objective: The goal of the trial was to compare a high-intensity intervention involving up-titration of heart failure (HF) treatments versus usual care among participants with admission for acute HF.

Study design: The STRONG-HF trial was a multinational, open-label, randomized, parallel-group trial of participants admitted with acute heart failure not on full doses of HF guideline-directed medical therapy

(GDMT). Patients were randomized in a 1:1 fashion to high-intensity uptitration ($n = 542$) or usual care ($n = 536$). Participants were stratified by left ventricular ejection fraction (LVEF) ($\leq 40\%$ vs. $>40\%$).

High-intensity care involved uptitration of treatments to 100% of recommended doses within 2 weeks of discharge for beta-blockers, angiotensin converting enzyme inhibitors (ACEIs) [or angiotensin receptor blockers (ARBs) if the patient was intolerant to ACEIs] or angiotensin receptor-neprilysin inhibitors, and mineralocorticoid receptor antagonists, and four scheduled outpatient visits over the 2 months after discharge with monitoring of clinical status, N-terminal pro–B-type natriuretic peptide (NT-proBNP) levels, and laboratory values.

The study was stopped early per Data and Safety Monitoring Board recommendation because of greater than expected between-group differences.

- *Total patients screened*: 1,641
- *Total randomized participants*: 1,078
- Study terminated on September 23, 2022
- *Mean patient age*: 63 years
- *Percentage female*: 39%
- *Percentage Black*: 21%

Inclusion criteria:
- Age 18–85 years
- Admission within 72 hours before screening for acute HF
- Hemodynamically stable
- NT-proBNP >2,500 pg/mL and >10% decrease between screening and before randomization (but still >1,500 pg/mL)
- Without treatment of optimal doses of oral HF therapies within 2 days before hospital discharge

Exclusion criteria: Intolerance to beta-blockers, ACEIs, or ARBs

Other salient features/characteristics:
- 29% with acute coronary syndrome
- 29% with diabetes
- 22% with New York Heart Association (NYHA) class IV HF 1 month before hospital admission
- 15% with left ventricular ejection fraction (LVEF) $\geq 50\%$
- *Baseline LVEF*: 36%
- *Cardiac resynchronization therapy (CRT) at baseline*: 1%

Result: The primary outcome, first occurrence of all-cause death or HF readmission by day 180, for the high-intensity care group versus usual care group, was 15.2% versus 23.3% ($p = 0.0021$).

The secondary outcome for high-intensity care group versus usual care group:
- All-cause death or HF readmission by day 90: 10.4% versus 13.8% ($p = 0.08$)
- All-cause death by day 180: 8.5% versus 10.0% ($p = 0.42$)
- Change in baseline to day 90 EQ-5D visual analog scale: 0.88 versus 0.90 ($p < 0.0001$)
- HF readmission by day 180: 9.5% versus 17.1% ($p = 0.0011$)
- Adjusted mean change in systolic blood pressure by day 90: –3.7 versus 1.6 mm Hg ($p < 0.0001$)
- Adjusted mean change in body weight by day 90: –1.78 versus –0.42 kg ($p < 0.0001$)
- Adjusted ratio of geometric mean of NT-proBNP: 0.44 versus 0.56 ($p = 0.0003$)

> **Key messages**
> - The STRONG-HF trial showed that, among patients with admission for acute HF, an intensive treatment strategy of rapid up-titration of guideline-directed medication reduced the risk recurrent hospitalization and all-cause death compared to usual care.
> - STRONG-HF was initiated prior to approval of SGLT-2Is for treatment of HF, and this medication class was mostly not used in this trial. Findings of this study give a clear message of benefit with early use of SGLT-2I in acute HF.

ARTICLE 12

Patiromer for the Management of Hyperkalemia in Heart Failure with Reduced Ejection Fraction: The DIAMOND Trial

Butler J, Anker SD, Lund LH, Coats AJS, Filippatos G, Siddiqi TJ, et al. Patiromer for the management of hyperkalemia in heart failure with reduced ejection fraction: the DIAMOND trial.
Eur Heart J. 2022;43(41):4362-73.

Abstract

Aim: In patients with heart failure with reduced ejection fraction (HFrEF), this present study is designed to inspect the influence of patiromer on the serum potassium level and its ability to enable specified use of target doses of renin–angiotensin–aldosterone system inhibitor (RAASI).

Methods and results: A total of 1,642 HFrEF patients were screened for current or a history of RAASi-related hyperkalemia and after screening 1,195 were registered in the run-in phase with patiromer and optimization of the RAASi therapy [≥50% suggested dose of angiotensin-converting enzyme inhibitor/angiotensin receptor blocker/angiotensin receptor-neprilysin inhibitor, and 50 mg of mineralocorticoid receptor antagonist (MRA) spironolactone or eplerenone]. In 878 (84.6%) patients, specified target doses of the RAASi therapy were attained; 439 were randomized to patiromer and 439 to placebo. All patients, physicians, and outcome assessors were blinded to treatment assignment. Obtaining observation between-group difference in the adjusted mean change in serum potassium was the primary endpoint of study. Here, assessed mainly five hierarchical secondary endpoints for the study. The median (interquartile range) duration of follow-up was 27 (13–43) weeks at the end of treatment, the adjusted mean change in potassium was +0.03 mmol/L in the patiromer group and +0.13 mmol/L in the placebo group {difference in the adjusted mean change between patiromer and placebo: −0.10 mmol/L [95% confidence interval (CI) −0.13, 0.07]; $p < 0.001$]}. With patiromer observed lower risk of hyperkalemia >5.5 mmol/L [hazard ratio (HR) 0.63; 95% CI 0.45, 0.87; $p = 0.006$], reduction of MRA dose (HR 0.62; 95% CI 0.45, 0.87; $p = 0.006$), and total adjusted hyperkalemia events/100 person-years (77.7 vs. 118.2; HR 0.66; 95% CI 0.53, 0.81; $p < 0.001$). Hyperkalemia-related morbidity-adjusted events (win ratio 1.53, $p < 0.001$) and total RAASI use score (win ratio 1.25, $p = 0.048$) favored the patiromer arm. Also, observed similar adverse events between groups.

Conclusion: The risk of recurrent hyperkalemia was reduced by concurrent use of patiromer and high-dose MRAs.

ARTICLE COMMENTARY

Objective: The goal of the trial was to evaluate patiromer compared with control among patients with heart failure with reduced ejection fraction (HFrEF) and history of hyperkalemia.

Study design:
- Randomized
- Parallel

Patients with HFrEF and hyperkalemia were randomized to patiromer ($n = 439$) versus control ($n = 439$). Prior to randomization, eligible patients had a run-in phase during which time patiromer was started, angiotensin-converting enzyme inhibitor/angiotensin receptor blocker/angiotensin receptor–neprilysin inhibitor optimized, and mineralocorticoid receptor antagonist (MRA) initiated/optimized. After the run-in phase, patients were randomized to continue patiromer versus stop patiromer.
- *Total number of enrollees:* 878
- *Duration of follow-up:* 13 weeks
- *Mean patient age:* 67 years
- *Percentage female:* 26%
- *Percentage with diabetes:* 42%

Inclusion criteria:
- HFrEF (left ventricular ejection fraction ≤40%)
- New York Heart Association class II–IV symptoms
- On beta-blocker or unable to tolerate beta-blocker
- Current or history of hyperkalemia

Exclusion criteria:
- Acute decompensated HF
- Estimated glomerular filtration rate <30 mL/min/1.73 m^2
- Systolic blood pressure <90 mm Hg
- Major cardiovascular event within the last 4 weeks

Other salient features/characteristics:
- Mean serum potassium: 4.6 mEq/L
- During the run-in phase, 85% of participants were able to be optimized on guideline-directed doses of renin–angiotensin–aldosterone system inhibitors (RAASIs)

Result: The primary outcome, adjusted mean change in serum potassium from randomization to study end, was 0.03 mEq/L in the patiromer group versus 0.13 mEq/L in the control group ($p < 0.001$).

Secondary outcomes:
- *Serum potassium >5.5 mEq/L:* 13.9% in the patiromer group versus 19.4% in the control group ($p = 0.006$)
- *Reduction in MRA dose below target:* 13.9% in the patiromer group versus 18.9% in the control group ($p = 0.006$)
- *Hyperkalemia-related outcomes win-ratio:* Ratio 1.53 ($p < 0.001$)
- *RAASI use-score win-ratio:* Ratio 1.25 ($p = 0.048$)

Interpretation: Use of patiromer in HFrEF patients is associated with lower incidence of hyperkalemia compared to control. 85% of participants with HFrEF have proper optimization of guideline-directed medical doses of RAASI.

> **Key message**
>
> - Hyperkalemia is one of the most common barriers to uptitrate RAAS blockers in patients with heart failure, that barrier can be removed by patiromer with increase adherence to RAASI, an important component of GDMT in HFrEF.

ARTICLE 13

Tolvaptan Add-on Therapy and Its Effects on Efficacy Parameters and Outcomes in Patients Hospitalized with Heart Failure

Kansara T, Gandhi H, Majmundar M, Kumar A, Patel JA, Kokkirala A, et al. Tolvaptan add-on therapy and its effects on efficacy parameters and outcomes in patients hospitalized with heart failure.
Indian Heart J. 2022;74(1):40-4.

Abstract

Introduction: In patients hospitalized with acute heart failure (HF), even with the adequate use of diuretics and vasodilators, volume overload and congestion are the major causes of morbidity and mortality. Present study aimed to assess the additive effect of tolvaptan on efficacy parameters as well as outcomes in hospitalized patients with HF.

Methods: PubMed, EMBASE, Cochrane library, and Web of Science databases for randomized controlled trials that studied the effects of tolvaptan versus placebo in hospitalized patients with HF were systematically searched. Mortality, rehospitalization, and hospital parameters like dyspnea relief, change in weight, sodium, and creatinine, studies contain any of the following endpoints then studies were included for analysis.

Results: Data from 14 studies involving 5,945 patients were analyzed for the meta-analysis. The follow-up duration ranged from 30 days to 2 years. There was no difference in mortality and rehospitalization between tolvaptan and placebo groups. Dyspnea relief score of HF patients was better (Likert score) in tolvaptan group and mean reduction in weight observed in the first 48 hours (short-term). But, the mean difference in weight was not significant, at 7 days (medium-term). In tolvaptan group, serum sodium levels increased significantly. Among the two groups, there was no difference in creatinine levels.

Conclusion: Tolvaptan helps in short-term symptomatic dyspnea relief and weight reduction shown by the present meta-analysis, but no long-term benefits observed including reduction in mortality and rehospitalization.

ARTICLE COMMENTARY

Diuretics in patients hospitalized with heart failure—finding the right space for tolvaptan!

Patients hospitalized with acute heart failure (AHF) have persistent volume overload and congestion even after the guideline-directed use of diuretics and vasodilators which is a vital contributor to mortality and morbidity. Additional challenges to decongestion in AHF include renal dysfunction, electrolyte imbalance, and show a poor response to diuretics.

Tolvaptan is a selective V2 receptor antagonist with the advantage of selective water diuresis without affecting sodium and potassium excretion. It has generated a large body of clinical data over the past decade after the seminal EVEREST trial. Previous data suggested that tolvaptan as add-on therapy can help reduce bodyweight, increase serum sodium concentration, and helps improving dyspnea score. But the study did not differentiate between short-term, medium- and long-term outcomes.

This is updated meta-analysis to compare the efficacy of tolvaptan as an add-on therapy with standard diuretic therapy in patients hospitalized with AHF and estimating its effects on clinical outcomes, length of stay, rehospitalization, and mortality. It included 14 randomized trials with close to 6,000 patients with study duration up to 2 years. The outcomes were reported in a time-sensitive manner <48 hour (short-term), up to 7 days (medium term) and 30 days and beyond (long-term).

The study concluded that adding tolvaptan provides significant dyspnea relief by reducing the volume overload within 48 hours along with weight loss that was seen during the short-term period not lasting beyond a week. That was accompanied by an increase in sodium concentration in the tolvaptan group. There was no effect of tolvaptan in the rehospitalization rates, length of stay, and mortality between the two groups—the results are in line with the EVEREST study. There was no change in the creatinine between the two groups, proving that tolvaptan did not caused significant renal dysfunction and can be used to manage congestion in chronic kidney disease (CKD) patients, although no mortality benefit was observed. The major reason for lack of sustained weight loss could be the selective V2 antagonism provided by tolvaptan highlighting the pivotal role of V1a receptor antagonism. The aquaretic efficacy of tolvaptan correlates well with baseline urine osmolality and baseline glomerular filtration rate (GFR), which may explain the higher initial aquaresis and weight loss in the 12 early phases of AHF after therapy initiation.

The million dollar question is where does Tolvaptan stand now? Loop diuretics will continue to be dominant therapy in patients with AHF and volume overload. However, certain clinical scenarios such as nephrotic syndrome and hypoalbuminemia reduce the delivery of furosemide to the distal tubules and lead to therapy. Presence of several organic anions, uric acid, and acidosis may additionally hamper the diuretic delivery to distal nephron. Escalation of doses of diuretic therapy predisposes the patient for electrolyte derangement. Tolvaptan promotes sustained reflow and glomerular filtration rate without affecting Na^+ and/or K^+ excretion. Tolvaptan can be used as rescue agent to increase diuresis and reduce body weight in such patients. On the contrary, the encouraging results of acetazolamide in AHF with congestion in the randomized ADVOR trial have garnered much interest and drug is expected to be evaluated in further studies.

The major limitations of the meta-analysis were under-reported adverse events and varied dosage use of tolvaptan.

In a nutshell, in patients hospitalized for AHF with features of congestion, tolvaptan can be utilized as an add-on therapy for symptomatic dyspnea relief and initial reduction in weight in selected cases. However, this benefit is short-lived and there is no advantage in reducing rehospitalization rates, mortality, or as a means of sustained weight loss.

> **Key messages**
> - In acute HF patients, residual congestion may persist despite aggressive use of loop diuretics.
> - Tolvaptan can be added to provide short-term dyspnea relief and weight loss in patients refractory to loop diuretics with better results and less adverse effects.
> - But tolvaptan use does not provide any long-term benefits (hospitalization rates, duration of stay, and mortality).

ARTICLE 14

β3 Adrenergic Agonist Treatment in Chronic Pulmonary Hypertension Associated with Heart Failure (SPHERE-HF): A Double Blind, Placebo-controlled, Randomized Clinical Trial

García-Álvarez A, Blanco I, García-Lunar I, Jordà P, Rodriguez-Arias JJ, Fernández-Friera L, et al. β3 adrenergic agonist treatment in chronic pulmonary hypertension associated with heart failure (SPHERE-HF): A double blind, placebo-controlled, randomized clinical trial.
Eur J Heart Fail. 2023;25(3):373-85.

Abstract

Aim: An increasingly prevalent problem associated with left heart disease is pulmonary hypertension (PH), orphan of targeted therapies, and related to a poor prognosis, particularly when pre- and postcapillary PH combine. The present study aimed to evaluate effect of treatment with the selective β3 adrenoreceptor agonist mirabegron or can it improve outcomes in patients with combined pre- and post-capillary PH (CpcPH).

Methods and results: This is a multicentre, randomized, parallel, placebo-controlled clinical trial. Enrolled stable patients with CpcPH associated with symptomatic heart failure, in the β3 Adrenergic Agonist Treatment in Chronic Pulmonary Hypertension Secondary to Heart Failure (SPHERE-HF) trial. To receive mirabegron (50 mg daily, titrated till 200 mg daily, $n = 39$) or placebo ($n = 41$), a total of 80 patients were assigned for 16 weeks. 66 patients were selected for the main analysis and successfully completed the study protocol. The change in pulmonary vascular resistance (PVR) on right heart catheterization was the primary endpoint. The change in right ventricular (RV) ejection fraction by cardiac magnetic resonance or computed tomography, other hemodynamic variables, functional class, and quality of life are the secondary outcomes.

Results of the trial was negative for the primary outcome [placebo-corrected mean difference of 0.62 Wood units, 95% confidence interval (CI) −0.38, 1.61, $p = 0.218$]. A significant improvement in RV ejection fraction was observed as compared to placebo (placebo-corrected mean difference of 3.0%, 95% CI 0.4, 5.7%, $p = 0.026$), in patients receiving mirabegron without display any significant differences in other prespecified secondary outcomes.

Conclusion: To evaluate the potential benefit of β3 adrenergic agonists in PH, the first clinical trial is SPHERE-HF. The primary endpoint, in patients with CpcPH is that the trial was negative since mirabegron did not reduce PVR. A significant improvement was found in RV ejection fraction assessed by advanced cardiac imaging, without differences in functional class or quality of life on the prespecified secondary outcomes.

ARTICLE COMMENTARY

SPHERE-HF: Novel β3 adrenergic agonist in chronic pulmonary hypertension associated with heart failure.

Pulmonary hypertension (PH) develops in heart failure [including both reduced ejection fraction (EF) and preserved EF] can be seen in up to two-thirds cases and portends a poor prognosis. A fraction of these patients have an ominous combination of pre- and postcapillary PH (CPH) manifested by more severe vascular remodeling, elevated vascular resistance, and worse outcomes. But currently, approved therapies for PH associated with HF are lacking.

Experimental and animal studies have demonstrated beneficial effect of β3 adrenergic stimulation (β3AR) leading to vasodilatation, reverse LV remodeling, improvement in pulmonary and right ventricular hemodynamics. Mirabegron is a selective oral β3 adrenergic agonist approved for neurogenic bladder dysfunction and shown to be safe in HF with reduced EF in a phase I study.

SPHERE-HF study aimed to determine the effects of using β3 adrenergic agonist mirabegron to improve outcomes among patients with HF and combined pre-and postcapillary PH (CppcPH). In this multi-centre trial, 80 patients with HF and right heart catheterization proven CPH were randomized to mirabegron and placebo. Mirabegron was initiated at 50 mg daily and titrated to 200 mg daily by 16 weeks. Patients were required to stable—NYHA class II–III, on standard guideline-directed therapy, without any recent hospitalization and need for therapy escalation. Patients with acute coronary syndromes, recent CRT implantation, severe renal failure, hepatic failure, uncontrolled hypertension, sinus tachycardia, AF, severe lung disease, QTc interval >480 ms, and concomitant vasodilator use were excluded.

The primary endpoint of study was change in the pulmonary vascular resistance measured by right heart catheterization at 16 weeks while the secondary outcomes included changes in the right ventricle ejection fraction assessed by cardiac MRI or CT, other hemodynamic variables, NYHA functional class, 6-minute walk distance, Borg dyspnea score, NT-proBNP, and quality of life. The researchers hypothesized that treatment with mirabegron in patients with CPH would result in beneficial effects due to reduction the PVR, increase in the RV performance, and improvement in clinical status without any serious adverse events.

Demographic and clinical characteristic at the baseline were well matched between the two groups. The primary outcome, i.e., change in PVR from baseline was not different with mirabegron treatment compared to placebo (median change in PVR from baseline to 16 weeks—+0.09 WU and −0.71 WU in the mirabegron and placebo arms respectively; $p = 0.218$). In the secondary outcomes, RV ejection fraction improved significantly from baseline (placebo corrected change of 3.0%; $p = 0.02$). There was no significant improvement in functional class and quality of life. No significant adverse effects related to the drug were seen either. Interestingly, the drug did not affect heart rate, systolic blood pressure, or oxygen saturation also.

The major limitations of notice of the trial were that heterogeneous cohorts of HFrEF and HFpEF were included and focusing on a single phenotype would have been more appropriate. Additionally, the use of thermodilution method for cardiac output calculation may be erroneous patients with severe TR which was present in many cases. Lastly, AF was evident in >70% cases which may have negated some of the beneficial effects of drugs.

In conclusion, mirabegron may have not achieved the primary outcome but significant improvement in RV ejection fraction can be ignored and needs to be explored further in a targeted and well-designed study.

Key messages

- Pulmonary hypertension in left heart failure carries poor prognosis and has no treatment available with significant benefits.
- Mirabegron, a selective β3 adrenergic agonist, has been used in SPHERE-HF in HF and catheterization-proven CPH with an aim to improve the PVR and other functional parameters.
- At 16 weeks, therapy with mirabegron did not show a decrease in PVR (primary goal) but there was improvement RV ejection fraction (secondary goal). The drug was well tolerated without any major safety signal.

ARTICLE 15

Effects of Sildenafil on Symptoms and Exercise Capacity for Heart Failure with Reduced Ejection Fraction and Pulmonary Hypertension (The SilHF Study): A Randomized Placebo Controlled Multicentre Trial

Cooper TJ, Cleland JGF, Guazzi M, Pellicori P, Ben Gal T, Amir O, et al. Effects of sildenafil on symptoms and exercise capacity for heart failure with reduced ejection fraction and pulmonary hypertension (the SilHF study): a randomized placebo-controlled multicentre trial.
Eur J Heart Fail. 2022;24(7):1239-48.

Abstract

Aim: Heart failure with reduced ejection fraction (HFrEF) complicated by pulmonary hypertension (PHT) and is associated with a substantial symptom burden and poor prognosis. Beneficial effects on pulmonary hemodynamics, cardiac function, and exercise capacity in HFrEF and PHT noted on using of sildenafil, a phosphodiesterase-5 (PDE-5) inhibitor. The aim of this present study was to evaluate the safety, tolerability, and efficacy of sildenafil in patients with HFrEF and indirect evidence of PHT.

Methods and results: An investigator-led, randomized, multinational trial is the Sildenafil in Heart Failure (SilHF) trial in which patients with HFrEF and a pulmonary artery systolic pressure (PASP) ≥40 mm Hg by echocardiography were randomly allocated in a 2:1 ratio to receive sildenafil (up to 40 mg three times/day) or placebo. Improvement in patient global assessment by visual analog scale and in the 6-minute walk test at 24 weeks was the co-primary endpoints of the study. Initially the sample size decided was 210 participants but, due to difficulties with supplying sildenafil/placebo and recruitment, only 69 patients were included {11 women, median age 68 years [interquartile range (IQR)] 62–74}, with median left ventricular ejection fraction 29% [IQR 24–35), median PASP 45 (IQR 42–55) mm Hg]. Sildenafil did not improve symptoms, quality of life, PASP, or walk test distance when compared to placebo. Those who were assigned to sildenafil had numerically more serious adverse events (33% vs. 21%), instead the sildenafil was generally well tolerated.

Conclusion: Sildenafil did not improve symptoms, quality of life, or exercise capacity in patients with HFrEF and PHT when compared to placebo.

ARTICLE COMMENTARY

Phosphodiesterase inhibition on heart failure—still a long way to go!

Pulmonary hypertension (PH) is not uncommon across the heart failure (HF) and the etiology is multifactorial including passive LA pressure, vasoconstriction, diminished compliance, and endothelial dysfunction. Phosphodiesterase-5 inhibition ameliorates endothelial dysfunction by replenishing the nitric oxide levels and this in turn is due to diminution of cyclic guanosine-3',5'-monophosphate (GMP) degradation. These drugs are a potent form of therapy for group 1 pulmonary hypertension but their role for PH in the setting of HF is unclear. Results of prior small and single center studies have been inconclusive. The *SilHF* was multicenter and placebo controlled study to investigate the effect of sildenafil on exercise capacity and symptoms in chronic HF with reduced ejection fraction complicated with PH.

In this investigator initiated study, 69 patients with HF with reduced EF [left ventricular ejection fraction (LVEF) <40%], NYHA Class II–III and echocardiography-defined PH (pulmonary artery systolic pressure >40 mm Hg) were enrolled. Additionally patients were required to have N-terminal proB-type natriuretic peptide (NTproBNP) >400 pg/mL or BNP >100 pg/mL, 6-minute walk distance (6MWD) <475 m and guideline-directed medical therapy for >3 months. Patients with acute coronary syndrome, prior hospitalization for HF, severe valvular heart disease, estimated glomerular filtration rate (eGFR) <40 mL/min, severe angina and uncontrolled

HTN (BP >160/90 mm Hg), and severe lung disease were excluded. Patients were randomized to sildenafil and placebo in 2:1 manner. Sildenafil was started at 10 mg once daily and rapidly uptitrated to 40 mg thrice daily in a fortnight. The primary endpoints were change in 6MWD and global symptom assessment by visual analog scale (VAS) score (EuroQol-5D). Change in NYHA class, quality of life assessed by KCCQ and EuroQol-5D, pulmonary artery systolic pressure (PASP) on echocardiography, renal function, safety and tolerability of drug were secondary endpoints.

At 24 weeks, there was no difference in 6MWD between both arms (+33 and +24 in placebo and sildenafil arms respectively; $p = 0.87$). Simultaneously, change in VAS score (EuroQol-5D) was also not different between two arms (+4.3 vs. +2.9 in placebo and sildenafil arms respectively; $p = 0.72$). There was similarly no difference in any other secondary endpoints either including PASP on echocardiography. Incidence of serious adverse effects was numerically higher with sildenafil but not statistically significant. Temporary therapy withdrawal was more common in sildenafil arm. Deaths were higher in sildenafil arm but again did not meet statistical significance.

Does this mean the end of road for sildenafil/phosphodiesterase-5 (PDE-5) inhibitors in HF? We do not know the answer yet. First, the trial initially planned to enroll 210 participants but did manage only 69 which led to trial being underpowered. The trail was interrupted for 18 months but fortunately, the researchers were able to complete it finally. Second, right heart catheterization was not performed for diagnosis of PH which is the gold standard for diagnosis. Third, unusually almost one-half of study population (46%) had permanent atrial fibrillation (AF). AF can lead to elevated LA pressures, poor quality of life, and morbidity independent of HF or PH. Fourth, the trial was not driven by clinical endpoints. It remains **Speculative that the Sildenafil would have been beneficial in patients of HFpEF if the study adequately Powered**. But, we would have been able to draw some meaningful conclusions regarding PDE-5 inhibition nevertheless. In fact, that would have been the largest trial of PDE-5I in HF with reduced EF till date. However, it is worthwhile to note that results of PDE-5 inhibitors in HF with preserved EF *(RELAX HF)* and Vericiguat (another vasodilator increasing NO) in HF with preserved EF *(SOCRATES PRESERVED)* were dismal.

Key messages

- The SilHF was a multicenter placebo-controlled randomized trial (n = 69) to evaluate the efficacy of sildenafil on symptoms and exercise capacity in patients with HF with reduced EF and PH.
- At 6 months, sildenafil neither produced improvement in any primary end points—6MWD or VAS score (EQ-5D) nor produced any beneficial effects in secondary end points—quality of life scores and echocardiographic parameters.
- Side effects and drug withdrawal were more frequent in sildenafil arm.

ARTICLE 16

Empagliflozin in Acute Myocardial Infarction: The EMMY Trial

Von Lewinski D, Kolesnik E, Tripolt NJ, Pferschy PN, Benedikt M, Wallner M, et al. Empagliflozin in acute myocardial infarction: the EMMY trial.
Eur Heart J. 2022;43(41):4421-32.

Abstract

Aim: The risk of hospitalization for heart failure and for death in patients with symptomatic heart failure is reduced by inhibition of sodium-glucose cotransporter-2. Still, evidence is lacking for the trials investigating the effects of this drug class in patients following acute myocardial infarction.

Methods and results: A total of $n = 476$ patients with acute myocardial infarction accompanied by a large creatine kinase elevation (>800 IU/L) were randomly assigned to empagliflozin 10 mg or matching placebo once daily within 72 hours of percutaneous coronary intervention in this academic, multicentre, double-blind trial. The N-terminal pro-hormone of brain natriuretic peptide (NT-proBNP) change over 26 weeks was the primary outcome. Changes in echocardiographic parameters are the included secondary outcomes. NT-proBNP was 1,294 (757–2,246) pg/mL was the baseline median (interquartile range). In the empagliflozin group, NT-proBNP reduction was significantly greater, compared with placebo, after adjusting for baseline NT-proBNP, sex, and diabetes status ($p = 0.026$) being 15% lower [95% confidence interval (CI) −4.4% to −23.6%]. A significant greater absolute left-ventricular ejection fraction improvement was observed (1.5%, 95% CI 0.2–2.9%, $p = 0.029$), mean E/e' reduction was 6.8% (95% CI 1.3–11.3%, $p = 0.015$) greater, and left-ventricular end-systolic and end-diastolic volumes were lower by 7.5 mL (95% CI 3.4–11.5 mL, $p = 0.0003$) and 9.7 mL (95% CI 3.7–15.7 mL, $p = 0.0015$), respectively, in the empagliflozin group, compared with placebo. For heart failure, seven patients were hospitalized (three in the empagliflozin group). Noted rare other predefined serious adverse events and between groups did not differ significantly.

Conclusion: Empagliflozin was associated with a significantly greater NT-proBNP reduction over 26 weeks in patients with a recent myocardial infarction, supplemented by a significant improvement in echocardiographic functional and structural parameters.

ARTICLE COMMENTARY

Sodium-glucose cotransporter-2 inhibitors (SGLT2-Is) inhibitors following acute MI—*Empagliflozin wins an Emmy*!

Sodium-glucose cotransporter-2 inhibitors are now advocated as one of the foundational pillars of optimal medical therapy for heart failure (HF) with both reduced and preserved ejection fraction (EF). Though, initially developed as antidiabetic drugs, the pivotal trials in diabetes mellitus had revealed significant reductions in hospitalization for HF (HHF). Subsequently, dedicated trials in HF with reduced EF and then preserved EF have revealed significant reductions in HHF and cardiovascular (CV) mortality.

Post-myocardial infarction (MI) period is a high-risk zone with poor ejection fraction and increased rates of incident heart failure. Despite optimal medical treatment and revascularization, event rates at follow-up continue to be high. SGLT-2I exhibits multiple cardioprotective effects and the benefits appear early after initiation of therapy. This provides a window of opportunity for its discharge in post-MI patients in preventing future HF events. The EMpagliflozin in patients with acute MYocardial infarction *(EMMY)* trial sought to evaluate the safety and efficacy of empagliflozin use over and above standard therapy in patients with large MI following revascularization.

In this prospective multicenter trial, 476 patients diagnosed with acute MI were enrolled within 72 hours following percutaneous coronary intervention (PCI) over a period of 5 years. Large MIs were defined based on elevated CPK-MB or Hs Troponin-T levels. Patients were randomized to empagliflozin 10 mg daily versus matching placebo for 26 weeks. Patients with type 1 diabetes mellitus, active urogenital infections, and prior SGLT-2I use were the main exclusions. The change in plasma NT-proBNP from baseline at week 26 was the main outcome. Improvement in echocardiographic parameters such as left ventricular ejection fraction (LVEF), left ventricle end-systolic dimension (LVESD), left ventricular end-diastolic volume (LVEDV), and diastolic function (E/e′) was the main secondary outcome measure. Multiple additional secondary outcome measures included change in NT-proBNP at week 6, change in body weight, and change in HbA1c.

At the trial completion, NT-proBNP decline was significantly higher by 15% in empagliflozin arm compared to placebo after adjustment ($p = 0.026$). The positive trend was significant by 12 weeks and the results remained significant after imputing the missing data in a sensitivity analysis. LVEF improvement was higher in the empagliflozin arm by an absolute 1.5% while E/e′ declined by 6.8%. LVEDV and LVESV were significantly smaller in intervention arm. Weight loss was again higher in the drug arm but without any marked change in HbA1c. Ketone body concentrations were higher in the SGLT-2I arm which has a mechanistic explanation. There was no difference in adverse events between both arms.

The NT-proBNP is a marker of left ventricular stress, future cardiovascular events and attenuation of plasma levels have been shown to be of prognostic significance. Thus, the encouraging results of EMMY trial are a hope in the direction of ameliorating events in the post-MI scenario. This also assumes significance in wake of dismal results from PARADISE-MI study wherein early initiation of angiotensin receptor–neprilysin inhibitor (ARNI) following MI failed to achieve significant reduction in major adverse cardiac event (MACE). Decline in natriuretic peptides was accompanied by improvements in LVEF, LV volumes, and diastolic function which can contribute to reverse remodeling and can have prognostic significance. It was a contemporary randomized controlled trial (RCT) with high usage of guideline-directed medical therapy (GDMT) (>95%) including RAAS blockers, beta-blockers, dual antiplatelet therapy, and statin adding to its strength. But the small sample size precluded any power to evaluate cardiovascular outcomes. Whether the beneficial effects seen in EMMY will translate into clinical outcome is being evaluated in two large CV outcome trials—EMPACT-MI (NCT04509674) and DAPA-MI (NCT04564742).

SECTION 5: Drug Therapy in Heart Failure

Key messages

- In EMMY trial, empagliflozin initiated within 72 hours of acute MI lead to a greater significant decline in NT-proBNP compared to placebo at 26 weeks.
- This was accompanied by increase in LVEF, decrease in LV volumes, and improvement in diastolic function.
- There were no safety issues but the trial was not powered for clinical/hard endpoints.

SECTION 6

Cardiomyopathy

Section Editor: **Sameer Dani**

Co-Editors: Mahpaekar Mashhadi, Bhuwan Chand Tewari

ARTICLE 1

Dose-blinded Myosin Inhibition in Patients with Obstructive Hypertrophic Cardiomyopathy Referred for Septal Reduction Therapy: Outcomes through 32 Weeks

Desai MY, Owens A, Geske JB, Wolski K, Saberi S, Wang A, et al. Dose-Blinded Myosin Inhibition in Patients With Obstructive Hypertrophic Cardiomyopathy Referred for Septal Reduction Therapy: Outcomes Through 32 Weeks. *Circulation. 2023;147(11):850-63.*

Abstract

Background: Patients of obstructive hypertrophic cardiomyopathy (oHCM), with intractable symptoms, have significant burden of mortality and morbidity with septal reduction therapy (SRT). VALOR-HCM trial evaluated the role of 32 weeks of mavacamten therapy in reducing the need for SRT.

Methods: It is a multicenter randomized double-blind trial that recruited patients of oHCM with left ventricular outflow tract (LVOT) gradients at rest or on provocation of ≥50 mm Hg between July 2020 and October 2021 from multiple US sites. These patients were on maximum medical therapy and electively planned for SRT. They received either continued mavacamten therapy for 32 weeks or placebo initially followed by mavacamten from 16th to 32 weeks of follow-up. Patients were later evaluated for LVOT gradients and LV ejection fraction (LVEF). The study of primary endpoint was to look for decline needs for SRT in both the groups of patients after 32 weeks.

Results: A total of 112 randomized patients with oHCM were enrolled, of which 108 qualified for study analysis (56 in mavacamten group and 52 in the placebo group) with mean age of 60.3 years and majority in either New York Heart Association (NYHA) class III or IV.

At completion of 32 weeks, 10.7% patients underwent SRT in mavacamten group and 13.5% in the placebo group. There was a continued decline in resting LVOT gradients and Valsalva gradients in the mavacamten group and similar reduction was observed in placebo cross over group. The NYHA class improved by 1 level in 90.6% of patients in mavacamten group and 70% of patients in placebo group.

Conclusion: Mavacamten treatment for 32 weeks showed a sustained reduction in the proportion proceeding to SRT, in severely symptomatic patients with oHCM, and effects were similar in placebo cross over group also.

ARTICLE COMMENTARY

In VALOR-HCM trial symptomatic adult patients with HOCM, for whom septal reduction therapy was planned, were subjected to either 32 weeks of continued *mavacamten* therapy or placebo followed by mavacamten from 16 weeks onward. Selective allosteric inhibitor of cardiac myosin ATPase *mavacamten* reduces cardiac actin-myosin cross-linking and attenuates contractility, improving compliance and energetics.

It is a multicenter randomized trial doubly blinded that recruited symptomatic obstructive hypertrophic cardiomyopathy (oHCM) patients with maximum tolerated doses of guideline-directed medical therapy (GDMT) referred for septal reduction therapy (SRT) between July 2020 and October 2021.

Major inclusion criteria:
- Patients referred for SRT with age >18 years
- Severe dyspnea or chest pain with maximum tolerated GDMT [New York Heart Association (NYHA) III/IV]
- Exertional syncope with NYHA-II
- Septal thickness ≥15 mm or 13 mm with family history of HCM
- Left ventricular outflow tract (LVOT) gradients (rest or on provocation) ≥50 mm Hg
- Left ventricular ejection fraction (LVEF) ≥60%

Major exclusion criteria:
- Did not meet SRT-guideline eligibility
- Not actively considering SRT
- LVEF < 60%
- Known infiltrative or storage disease as a cause of HOCM
- Not on a stable dose of medication
- Did not hold prohibitory medications for 14 days
- Paroxysmal AF without adequate rate control or anticoagulation
- Aortic stenosis
- Coronavirus disease 2019 (COVID-19) infection in the past 90 days
- Withdrawal by subject

The study was designed and sponsored by Cleveland Clinic Coordinating Center for Clinical Research, and Medpace, and was reviewed by internal boards at centers, recruiting patients that consented. The study was funded by MyoKardia, Inc, a wholly-owned subsidiary of Bristol Myers Squibb.

Initially, 112 patients were randomized 1:1 manner to placebo and mavacamten (5 mg/day). Echocardiographic follow-up was done every 4 weeks to adjust the dose of mavacamten. At the 16th week, patients originally subjected to a placebo were crossed over to mavacamten 5 mg/day. Two groups have identical baseline demographic and hemodynamic properties by echocardiography. In the patients with LVEF < 50% at any point of time with mavacamten on, the therapy was withheld for 4 weeks and started with LVEF > 50% on follow-up with dose 1 level below the last dose. If LVEF falls below 30% at any point in time, the therapy is permanently stopped.

On completion of 32 weeks follow-up, only 10.7% in mavacamten group and 13.5% in the placebo cross-over group, required SRT as per guideline criteria. Further a sustained decline in both resting and provocative LVOT gradients were observed in mavacamten group as well in placebo cross-over group. 90.6% patients in the mavacamten group and 70% in the cross-over group showed improvement of at least 1 level in their NYHA class. The benefits were sustained over the period of time till 36 weeks in both groups.

Limitation: Small sample size and shorter duration of study could not provide adequate data regarding safety outcomes and long-term mortality benefits, if any with the *mavacamten* therapy. The study includes the white population largely. It was a pharma-funded study.

CONCLUSION

There was a significant reduction in LVOT gradients, NYHA class, cardiac biomarkers, and KCCQ-23-CSS with the institution of the mavacamten therapy in both the original mavacamten group and the cross-over placebo group. Mavacamten seems probable alternative for those oHCM patients who are on maximum guideline-directed medical therapy while awaiting for SRT.

ARTICLE 2

Survival Following Alcohol Septal Ablation or Septal Myectomy for Patients with Obstructive Hypertrophic Cardiomyopathy

Cui H, Schaff HV, Wang S, Lahr BD, Rowin EJ, Rastegar H, et al. Survival Following Alcohol Septal Ablation or Septal Myectomy for Patients With Obstructive Hypertrophic Cardiomyopathy.
J Am Coll Cardiol. 2022;79(17):1647-55.

Abstract

Background: The long-term mortality outcomes comparing alcohol septal ablation (ASA) with septal myectomy remain unclear due scarcity of available trail data.

Objectives: This study compares primary endpoint of long-term mortality with ASA versus septal myectomy in obstructive hypertrophic cardiomyopathy (oHCM).

Methods: The study enrolled 3,859 patients undergoing either ASA or septal myectomy at selected specialized oHCM centers. The primary endpoint of the study was to investigate all-cause mortality.

Results: About 15.2% study patients underwent ASA and 84.8% underwent septal myectomy. The ASA group comprised older individuals with lesser septal thickness and higher prevalence of diabetes, hypertension, renal impairment, and coronary artery disease. Early mortality occurred in 0.7% patients of ASA and 0.3% patients of myectomy group. Further follow-up of 6.4 years revealed all-cause mortality of 26.15 with ASA and 8.2% with myectomy group. Ever after comorbidity adjusted, mortality remained higher with ASA.

Conclusion: In obstructive hypertrophic cardiomyopathy patients, it was observed that ASA is associated with increased long-term all-cause mortality when compared with septal myectomy, which was independent of existing confounding comorbidities as well.

ARTICLE COMMENTARY

There has been a long-standing controversy regarding the merits of septal myectomy versus alcohol septal ablation (ASA), no RCT (randomized controlled trial) data is available till now and meta-analysis of the observational studies so far suggests comparable early mortality in both procedures with a higher incidence of pacemaker implantation and residual left ventricular outflow tract (LVOT) gradient in ASA patients.

This study compared long-term mortality benefits in the patients who underwent septal reduction therapy in three high-volume-experienced centers (Minnesota, Boston, and Beijing).

This is a retrospective study with data from the centers for all septal reduction procedures (SRP) from 1998 to 2019. Patients who underwent concurrent cardiac surgery (CABG/valve replacement) or already had undergone SRP prior to the index procedure were excluded from the study. All-cause mortality was the primary outcome and survival data was obtained from the prospectively maintained database from the respective centers.

A total of 3,859 patients were included in the study, 3,274 patients had undergone myectomy, and 585 patients had ASA. When we look at demographic data and baseline characteristics of the patients, the mean age of the patients is higher in the ASA group and the mean septal thickness is higher in the myectomy group. ASA patients had relatively more comorbidities than the septal myectomy group.

After completion of median follow-up, the all-cause mortality in the ASA group was 26.1% and in the myectomy group, 8.2%. Multivariate adjustment also revealed higher mortality in ASA (HR 1.68; 95% CI 1.29–2.19; $p < 0.001$). Comparing of septal thickness, the results were similar between the two groups (interaction $p = 0.217$). The estimated mortality risk with ASA was worse among class IV NYHA (New York Heart Association) patients. The Kaplan Meir curve for mortality showed a similar risk of death with either procedure. The results may be due to a higher occurrence of complete heart block in the ASA patients and benefit of survival offered by potential surgical risk and quality of life.

Limitations: It is a retrospective study—might have some selection bias. Data regarding postprocedure complications and pacemaker implantation are not available. Data regarding the cause of death, whether cardiovascular or systemic illness was not available. ASA group had older patients with more comorbidities. Follow-up data about septal thickness and LVOT gradients are not available, as their reduction possibly takes a few months to appear effectiveness of the ASA cannot be commented upon.

Key message

- In oHCM, septal myectomy occurs long-term survival benefit over ASA, even when adjusting for other confounding factors and also promises to offer better quality of life.

ARTICLE 3

Systemic Embolism, a Dreaded Complication in Amyloid Transthyretin Cardiomyopathy

Vilches S, Fontana M, Gonzalez-Lopez E, Mitrani L, Saturi G, Renju M, et al. Systemic embolism in amyloid transthyretin cardiomyopathy.
Eur J Heart Fail. 2022;24(8):1387-96.

Abstract

Aims: Currently knowledge about the incidence and prevalence of systemic embolism in transthyretin amyloid cardiomyopathy (ATTR-CM) is limited. This study aimed to look into the incidence, prevalence, and associated factors of systemic embolization in ATTR-CM. Further, the role of oral anticoagulation (OAC) and use of the CHA_2DS_2-VASc score in such patients was also explored in this study.

Methods and results: It is a retrospective study enrolling patients with ATTR-CM at multiple international centers for amyloid. A total of 1,191 patients were recruited with ATTR-CM majority of wild-type transthyretin cardiac amyloidosis (ATTRwt type) with more representation of male population, with median age 77.1 years. Prior to study 13.6% had experience one or more embolic event. During follow-up of 19.9 months, 3.44% had an embolization. This incidence reported as per 100 patient-years was zero (the lowest) with OAC in sinus rhythm, 1.3 times without OAC in sinus rhythm, 1.7 with OAC in AF, and the highest as 4.8 without OAC in atrial fibrillation (AF). Embolic events risk was estimated by CHA_2DS_2-VASc. No difference was observed in the embolic events between AF patients treated with vitamin K antagonists (VKAs) and direct oral anticoagulants (DOACs) treated patients ($p = 0.66$).

Conclusion: The risk of systemic embolism is real in ATTR-CM and can be reduced significantly with OAC. Both VKAs and DOACs are effective as OAC. The CHA_2DS_2-VASc score correlates poorly with embolic events in ATTR-CM and hence cannot be used for profiling thromboembolic risk in this cohort.

ARTICLE COMMENTARY

Thromboembolic phenomenon because of atrial arrhythmias including atrial fibrillation (AF) and flutter is prevalent in high numbers in transthyretin amyloid cardiomyopathy (ATTR-CM) especially with its wild variant, ATTRwt.

This study was uniquely conducted to estimate the incidence and prevalence of these thromboembolic events in a large multicentric cohort of ATTR-CM. It also studied the utility of the CHA_2DS_2-VASc score in predicting thromboembolic events.

This multicentric longitudinal study enrolled cohort of adult ATTR-CM patients (ATTRv or ATTRwt) from four international centers for amyloid. ATTR-CM was said to be present when one of the following conditions was fulfilled: (1) Biopsy results from endomyocardium suggestive of TTR amyloid, or (2) Extracardiac biopsy with evidence for

TTR amyloid deposits and further presence of one or more of the following: (i) on echocardiogram, unexplained increased left ventricular (LV) wall thickness ≥12 mm; (ii) cardiac magnetic resonance (CMR) findings suggesting cardiac amyloidosis with diffuse gadolinium uptake; and (iii) photon emission computed tomography showing cardiac uptake grade 2 or 3, or (iii) single-photon emission computed tomography (SPECT) with cardiac uptake grade 2 or 3 and no monoclonal protein in CMR. Further, all these cases were confirmed with genetic testing for presence of *TTR* gene mutations.

Total 1,191 individuals of ATTR-CM majority with ATTRwt with 87.1% being males and median age of 77 years were enrolled. Of these 52.5% patients already had AF, 88.7% were receiving OAC, and 13.6% already had systemic embolization. In follow-up period of 19.9 months, 3.44% patients further developed embolic events. Among these 57.1% already had AF and 26% developed new onset of AF 16.7% neither had nor developed AF during follow-up. The prevalence of thromboembolism was 16.2%. This incidence rate was higher in those without AF not receiving OAC.

Exploring the incidence rates of thromboembolism in those with AF receiving OAC to those with AF without OAC, latter had the highest rates (4.8 per 100 patients). Applying CHA_2DS_2-VASc score, only those with score ≥3 had embolisms. In the non-AF cohort, three had CHA_2DS_2-VASc score 0–1 but suffered embolic phenomenon on follow-up. Thus, questioning the utility of CHA_2DS_2-VASc score. OAC patients survived better and there was no difference between incidence rates with VKA and DOACs.

■ CONCLUSION

Thromboembolic events remain the predominant complications in patients with ATTR-CM, with incidence rates as high as 16.2%. These events occur in patients with ATTR-CM irrespective of the presence of atrial fibrillation, with increased frequency in AF patients. CHA_2DS_2-VASc score turns out to be a poor predictor of thromboembolic events irrespective of the rhythm status of the patients. Vitamin K antagonists (VKAs) and DOACs are effective anticoagulants with insignificant differences in efficacy and bleeding risk. International Normalized Ratio (INR) should be maintained in the therapeutic range for patients on VKAs for optimal results.

ARTICLE 4

Structural and Functional Brain Changes in Acute Takotsubo Syndrome

Khan H, Gamble DT, Rudd A, Mezincescu AM, Abbas H, Noman A, et al. Structural and Functional Brain Changes in Acute Takotsubo Syndrome.
JACC Heart Fail. 2023;11(3):307-17.

Abstract

Background: An acute myocardial infarction mimicked by Takotsubo syndrome, characteristically in the aftermath of mental or physical stress.

Objectives: Currently, limited knowledge exists about the mechanism by which emotional processing in the context of stress leads to significant cardiac injury, so a detail exploration of brain structure and function in patients with takotsubo syndrome add merits to the analysis.

Methods: In this observational cross-sectional study, a total of 25 acute (<5 days) takotsubo patients and 25 control subjects were recruited. On magnetic resonance imaging (MRI) brain scans, surface-based morphometry was carried out to extract cortical morphology centered on volume, thickness, and surface area with the use of Freesurfer. For age, sex, photoperiod, and total brain volume, cortical morphology general linear models were corrected. Functional Magnetic Resonance Imaging of the Brain Diffusion Toolbox and Functional Connectivity Toolbox were used for resting-state functional MRI and diffusion tensor tractography images and were preprocessed and analyzed.

Results: Here observed statistically significant smaller total white matter and subcortical gray matter volumes in Takotsubo ($p < 0.001$), with smaller total brain surface area but increased total cortical thickness (both $p < 0.001$). In Takotsubo patients, individual gray matter regions (hippocampus and others) were significantly smaller ($p < 0.001$); only larger thalamus and insula ($p < 0.001$) were observed. In multiple areas, both significant hyperfunctional and hypofunctional connectivity were observed, which include thalamus-amygdala-insula and basal ganglia ($p < 0.05$). Increase in all structural tractography connections was seen in Takotsubo ($p < 0.05$) patients.

Conclusion: The authors revealed that smaller cortical surface area drove smaller gray and white matter volumes, but observed increased cortical thickness and structural tractography connections with bidirectional changes in functional connectivity linked to emotion, language, reasoning, perception, and autonomic control. These findings are interventional targets in rehabilitation of Takotsubo patients.

ARTICLE COMMENTARY

The article published in JACC by *Khan et al.*, titled Brain Changes in Acute Takotsubo Syndrome shows changes in brain structure, function, and structural connectivity in patients with acute Takotsubo syndrome, using MRI and functional MRI.

They studied 25 patients with acute Takotsubo syndrome and 25 controls, predominantly female (only one male) who were within 5 days of diagnosis. Among study subjects with acute Takotsubo syndrome, 40% of patients had emotional triggers, 28% had physical triggers and 32% had no obvious trigger. The mean LVEF was 45% ± 8.3%.

They meticulously did a psychological questionnaire assessment and environmental variable photoperiod analysis and found that anxiety and depression scales were significantly higher in the acute Takotsubo syndrome group.

MRI scans evaluated cortical surface areas and thickness, white matter hyperintensity volume, gray matter volume, structural connectivity using diffusion tensor imaging, and resting state connectivity using functional MRI showing significantly smaller cortical surface area in several brain regions, such as left rostral, anterior cingulate, right and left insula. At the same time, cortical thickness was higher, especially in the right insula among cases as compared to controls.

Acute Takotsubo patients had significantly smaller white matter and subcortical gray matter volumes, whereas their cortical gray matter was larger.

Their limbic system also showed significant differences.

Acute Takotsubo patients have smaller hippocampus and brainstem volumes but larger thalamus and insula volume as compared to matched controls.

Interestingly, although structural connectivity (on tractography) was significantly increased in acute Takotsubo syndrome patients (specific thalamus to the temporal regions, left insula to the right amygdala, right Putamen, right posterior cingulate gyrus, right rostral anterior cingulate gyrus), the functional connectivity was significantly decreased in the same areas.

The abnormal insular function as observed in this study, as well as some previous studies, suggests maladaptive response and abnormal function of the insular region could play a role in the pathogenesis of acute Takotsubo syndrome. This finding could support the "nitrosative theory" of acute Takotsubo syndrome, where there is a maladaptive brain response to stress involving the thalamus, amygdala, and insular pathways, leading to loss of autonomic control over the nervous system resulting in sympathetic overactivity which ultimately leads to myocardial injury, presenting as acute Takotsubo syndrome.

This observational study provides insight and is hypothesis-generating for further research. Follow-up MRI may help in clarifying the evolution of these central nervous system (CNS) abnormalities and identifying if there is any reversibility in these structural and functional abnormalities.

However, study has some limitations like a small sample size, having only one male patient, and lack of follow-up MRI to study the evolution of CNS changes. Despite these limitations, the study has provided a novel insight into the CNS abnormalities in these patients and enhanced knowledge in the field of heart-brain connections. The findings of this study may lead to further evaluation of therapeutic options acting on higher-level of CNS functional areas for Takotsubo patients.

ARTICLE 5

The Prevalence and Association of Exercise Test Abnormalities with Sudden Cardiac Death and Transplant-free Survival in Childhood Hypertrophic Cardiomyopathy

Conway J, Min S, Villa C, Weintraub RG, Nakano S, Godown J, et al. The Prevalence and Association of Exercise Test Abnormalities With Sudden Cardiac Death and Transplant-Free Survival in Childhood Hypertrophic Cardiomyopathy.
Circulation. 2023;147(9):718-27.

Abstract

Background: Abnormal exercise responses in hypertrophic cardiomyopathy (HCM) are predictors of heart failure and poor outcomes. This study aimed to evaluate an abnormal exercise response with outcomes in pediatric HCM population.

Methods: This study included 20 centers, enrolling phenotype-positive-primary HCM patients aged <18 years of age. Exercise response was defined abnormal if blunted blood pressure response and worsening ST- or T-wave segment changes were observed or complex ventricular ectopic occurred. Study defined sudden cardiac death (SCD) events as a composite of SCD and aborted sudden cardiac arrest.

Results: Around 630 patients underwent exercise testing with no significant difference in baseline clinical characteristics. The population median age was 13.8 years 78% males and 39% on β-blockers. A total of 28% abnormal test results were recorded. Abnormal test population showed higher left ventricular outflow tract (LVOT) gradients, higher values of z scores for left atrium diameter, more severe septal hypertrophy, and higher prevalence of myectomy compared with patients with normal test results ($p < 0.05$). Such abnormal response population were estimated with poor 5-year transplant-free survival ($p = 0.005$). Further those with inducible ischemia were estimated with higher odds for having all-cause death or transplant [hazard ratio (HR) 4.86), to be followed only by population with abnormal blood pressure response (HR 3.19). There were lower odds of SCD free survival period in those with inducible ischemia, but exercise ectopy was not associated with poor survival.

Conclusion: In childhood, HCM exercise abnormal exercise test results are markers of lower transplant-free survival, the lowest when response is inducible ischemia. There is also increased risk of SCD events. Despite all the available evidence, the routine exercise testing in childhood HCM remains a topic of debate.

ARTICLE COMMENTARY

The study by Jennifer Conway et al. is a multicentric retrospective study. The authors studied phenotype-positive-primary hypertrophic cardiomyopathy (HCM) patients who were younger than 18 years of age, and who underwent a treadmill or bicycle exercise stress test. A septal or posterior wall thickness >2 standard deviation was defined as a positive phenotype HCM. Cases with isolated HCM and no other cause for left ventricular hypertrophy (LVH) were labeled as primary HCM.

An abnormal exercise response was defined in study as either abnormal BP response with absence of rise in systolic BP by ≥20 mm Hg or a fall in systolic BP with exercise) along with ischemic ECG changes or occurrence of complex ventricular ectopics manifested as frequent single premature ventricular contractions or ventricular couplets or ventricular bigeminy, or consecutive three premature ventricular contractions, or their combination.

Overall, 7% of patients experienced aborted SCA, 1% experienced sudden cardiac death (SCD), 1% died from other causes, and 3% underwent a heart transplant on a 5-year follow-up. An implantable cardioverter defibrillator (ICD) insertion and appropriate ICD discharges were more frequent in those with abnormal exercise test results.

All-cause mortality or transplantation was more frequently associated with abnormal ST-T or ischemic response, while patients with ventricular ectopy did not experience any event.

Five years of freedom from SCD events was not different between those with normal versus abnormal exercise test results but on subgroup analysis, 5-year SCD event-free survival varied by type of abnormal exercise response. In those with the ischemic response, the rate of SCD was 5.89 events per 100 person-years compared with 1.7 events for those with an abnormal BP response and 1.41 events for those with normal exercise test results.

Abnormal response population had significantly higher cumulative 5-year proportion of death or transplant especially it was the highest in those with inducible ischemia. The SCD risk was also higher in such patients but exercise of ectopy was not associated with increased SCD risk.

In the index study, 28% of pediatric HCM patients had abnormal exercise test response, which was an independent predictor of lower transplant-free survival and all-cause mortality. A very important finding in this study was that worsening ST-T changes from baseline suggesting ischemia was most strongly associated with events whereas the exercise-induced ventricular ectopy was not a predictor of SCD.

The study highlights the importance of routine exercise stress testing in pediatric HCM patients for the risk stratification for SCD as well as progression to stage of frank heart failure. It also suggests that findings of myocardial ischemia during exercise stress tests may help in identifying pediatric HCM patients who are at high risk for life-threatening arrhythmia. Patients with abnormal exercise test responses had more SCD events, more ICD implantation, and more appropriate ICD shocks.

Though the potential limitations associated with retrospective study design, such as bias and confounding effects of practice variability cannot be totally ruled out, the careful design of the study suggests that these factors are less likely to be significant.

This study showed the utility of exercise testing in pediatric HCM patients as a risk assessment tool and to help in better-guiding treatment and prognostication.

SECTION 7

Arrhythmia and Heart Failure

Section Editor: Aditya Kapoor

Co-Editors: Deepchandh Raja, Daljeet Kaur Saggu, Muthiah Subramaniam, Anindya Ghosh

ARTICLE 1

Incidence of Sudden Cardiac Death and Life-threatening Arrhythmias in Clinically Manifest Cardiac Sarcoidosis with and without Current Indications for an Implantable Cardioverter Defibrillator

Nordenswan HK, Pöyhönen P, Lehtonen J, Ekström K, Uusitalo V, Niemelä M, et al. Incidence of Sudden Cardiac Death and Life-Threatening Arrhythmias in Clinically Manifest Cardiac Sarcoidosis With and Without Current Indications for an Implantable Cardioverter Defibrillator.
Circulation. 2022;146(13):964-75.

Abstract

Background: Cardiac sarcoidosis (CS) predisposes to sudden cardiac death (SCD). The Heart Rhythm Society (HRS) in 2014 and the American College of Cardiology/American Heart Association/HRS (ACC/AHA/HRS) consortium in 2017 have issued guidelines for implantable cardioverter defibrillators (ICDs) in CS. Discrimination strategies from high to low risk remain unclear.

Methods: The data of total 398 patients with CS observed in Finland from 1988 to 2017 were analyzed. All patients were presented with clinical cardiac manifestations. In 193 patients (definite CS), histological diagnosis was myocardial and extracardiac in 205 (probable CS). At presentation, patients with and without Class I or IIa ICD indications were identified, and subsequent manifestations of SCD (fatal or aborted) and sustained ventricular tachycardia were noted, who have ICD indications appeared first on follow-up.

Results: A total of 41 patients (10.3%) had fatal ($n = 8$) or aborted ($n = 33$) SCD, and 98 (24.6%) experienced SCD or sustained ventricular tachycardia as the first event, over a median of 4.8 years. On following the guideline given by the HRS, Class I or IIa ICD indications were found to be present in 339 patients (85%) and absent in 59 (15%), of whom 264 (78%) and 30 (51%), respectively, received an ICD. Presentation of cumulative 5-year incidence for SCD was observed 10.7% (95% CI 7.4–15.4%) in ICD indicated patients versus 4.8% (95% CI 1.2–19.1%) in those without ICD ($\chi^2 = 1.834$, $p = 0.176$). The corresponding rates of SCD were 13.8%

(95% CI 9.1–21.0%) versus 6.3% (95% CI 0.7–54.0%; $\chi^2 = 0.814$, $p = 0.367$) in definite CS and 7.6% (95% CI 3.8–15.1%) versus 3.3% (95% CI 0.5–22.9%; $\chi^2 = 0.680$, $p = 0.410$) in probable CS. SCD was anticipated by definite histological diagnosis ($p = 0.033$) but not by Class I or IIa ICD indications ($p = 0.210$) on applying multivariable regression analysis. At the time of presentation, patients without ICD indications, 5-year incidence of SCD, sustained ventricular tachycardia, and emerging Class I or IIa indications were noted, 53% (95% CI 40–71%). Guideline specified by the ACC/AHA/HRS indicated that all patients with complete data ($n = 245$) had Class I or IIa indications for ICD implantation.

Conclusion: Presently existing ICD guidelines fail to discriminate a truly low-risk group of patients with clinically manifest CS. But, the 5-year risk of SCD approaching 5% in spite of absent ICD indications. Hence, there is a necessity of future research on prognostic factors which include the role of diagnostic histology. For the meantime, all CS patients should be considered for an ICD implantation, presented with clinical cardiac expressions.

ARTICLE COMMENTARY

Prevention of sudden cardiac death (SCD) remains one of the greatest decision-making challenges in patients with cardiac sarcoidosis (CS). Nordenswan et al. analyzed the risk of SCD and ventricular arrhythmias (VAs) in patients with definite or probable CS. The authors selected subjects with CS from a (Myocardial Inflammatory Diseases in Finland) MIDFIN registry. They go through the data from two groups of the selected subjects, those with and without Class I or IIa indications for placement of an implantable cardioverter defibrillator (ICD), based on 2014 Heart Rhythm Society (HRS) consensus document. As expected, patients with Class I or IIa indication exhibited a 5-year cumulative event rate of 24% with SCD risk of 10%. Importantly, those without Class I or IIa indication exhibited a 5-year cumulative risk of 12% with a SCD risk of 5%. Within this group of 59 patients, 53% had progressive sarcoid cardiomyopathy and/or VAs during the follow-up period.

Even among CS patients with preserved left ventricular ejection fraction (LVEF), there is a significant risk of VAs and SCD. In just the first year after an abnormal cardiac magnetic resonance imaging finding with late gadolinium enhancement (CMRI-LGE) in patients with a preserved LVEF: The risk of aborted sudden death or appropriate ICD shocks was noted >20%. Quantitatively, a burden of LGE of >6% has been suggested as an appropriate cut-off point for the prediction of future arrhythmic events. From our institutional Granulomatous Myocarditis Registry, immunosuppression in patients with CS led to a significant reduction in the burden of VAs both in patients with and without LV dysfunction. Of 64 patients with biopsy-positive CS who presented with VAs, immunosuppression led to a reduction in VA burden in 56 patients (87.5%). Although this study was not powered to understand the effect of immunosuppressive therapy on SCD risk, the cardiac sarcoidosis multi-center randomized controlled trial (CHASM CS-RCT) is an ongoing trial that may shed more light on the effects of immunosuppressive therapy.

Some authors have investigated the utility of programmed electrical stimulation (PES) to recognize patients with CS at the highest risk of SCD. Although PES may be able to identify patients with CS with arrhythmic potential, it does not consider the potential for the progression of cardiac disease. In this regard, more than half of the patients with CS in this study exhibited progression of cardiac involvement during follow-up. These findings may expand way to explain condition of the lower but significant VA/SCD risk profile over 5 years, building strategy for early ICD implantation as a rational option.

The authors need to be congratulated for their significant contribution to CS literature. This data is in favor of an amendment of currently present guidelines addressing ICD indications for patients with CS. To discuss the benefits and risks patients with preserved LVEF and abnormal advanced imaging should be well-thought-out for ICD therapy through a common decision-making approach **(Box 1)**. Numerous questions remain for the most appropriate risk stratification and management strategies for patients with CS and preserved LVEF. Formulation of an international registry would seem to be an appropriate next step. The information gained from this registry would assist clinicians who manage patients with this challenging disease.

> **BOX 1** Proposed indications for primary prevention ICD in patients with cardiac sarcoidosis.
>
> - Sustained VT or cardiac arrest
> - LVEF < 35%
> - LVEF > 35% with syncope
> - LVEF > 35% with an indication for permanent pacing
> - LVEF > 35% with an estimated scar (CMR) > 10%
> - LVEF > 35% with an inducible ventricular arrhythmia
>
> (CMR: cardiovascular magnetic resonance; ICD: implantable cardioverter-defibrillator; LVEF: left ventricular ejection fraction; VT: ventricular tachycardia)

ARTICLE 2

Randomized Trial of Left Bundle Branch versus Biventricular Pacing for Cardiac Resynchronization Therapy

Wang Y, Zhu H, Hou X, Wang Z, Zou F, Qian Z, et al. Randomized Trial of Left Bundle Branch vs Biventricular Pacing for Cardiac Resynchronization Therapy.
J Am Coll Cardiol. 2022;80(13):1205-16.

Abstract

Background: The most rapidly emergent conduction system pacing technique, left bundle branch pacing (LBBP) is widely used for correcting intrinsic left bundle branch block (LBBB). Subsequently, it is definitely an ideal alternative to cardiac resynchronization therapy (CRT) with biventricular pacing (BiVP).

Objectives: Authors aimed to compare the efficacy of LBBP-CRT with BiVP-CRT in heart failure patients and reduced left ventricular ejection fraction (LVEF).

Methods: Present study is a prospective, randomized trial of patients presented with nonischemic cardiomyopathy and LBBB with 6-month preplanned follow-up. If LBBP or BiVP was unsuccessful then crossovers were permissible. The primary goal was to recognize the difference in LVEF improvement among two groups. The secondary goal involved measurements of changes in echocardiograph, N-terminal pro–B-type natriuretic peptide (NT-proBNP), New York Heart Association (NYHA) functional class, 6-minute walk distance, (6MWD) QRS duration, and CRT response.

Results: Present study included a total of 40 consecutive patients (20 males, mean age 63.7 years, LVEF 29.7% ± 5.6%). Observed crossovers in 10% of LBBP-CRT and 20% of BiVP-CRT. All patients are regularly followed up. Significantly higher LVEF improvement at 6 months after LBBP-CRT than BiVP-CRT (mean difference: 5.6%; 95% CI 0.3–10.9; $p = 0.039$) indicated by intention-to-treat analysis. LBBP-CRT also emerges to show a greater reduction in left ventricular end-systolic volume (−24.97 mL; 95% CI −49.58 to −0.36 mL) and NT-proBNP (−1,071.80 pg/mL; 95% CI −2,099.40 to −44.20 pg/mL), and comparable changes in NYHA functional class, 6MWD, QRS duration, and rates of CRT response compared with BiVP-CRT.

Conclusion: LBBP-CRT revealed promising LVEF improvement than BiVP-CRT with nonischemic cardiomyopathy and LBBB in heart failure patients.

ARTICLE COMMENTARY

Physicians search for the most physiologic pacing for both bradyarrhythmias and heart failure (HF) with wide QRS has led to the rapid evolution of conduction system pacing (CSP) over the last decade. Thus, CSP and especially left bundle branch area pacing (LBBAP) is a rapidly evolving tool world over for both these indications. To date, there is no precise definition to differentiate left bundle pacing (LBP) from left ventricular septal pacing (LVSP) and left bundle fascicle pacing (LBFP) and there is no data to show major differences in the outcome among these sites of pacing. Thus, the terminology of LBBAP is widely accepted till we have long-term outcome data with randomized trials showing the difference in the outcome among these modalities of pacing.

There are a lot of small studies on the feasibility and outcome of LBBAP. Jastrzebski et al. have reported the largest feasibility and outcome data of LBBAP, performed across 14 European centers for both bradyarrhythmia and HF indication in lieu of biventricular pacing (BiVP). They precisely differentiated the criteria for LBP, LBFP (anterior fascicle, posterior fascicle, and septal fascicle), and LVSP. This study enrolled >2,500 patients across 14 centers and reported follow-up over 6.4 ± 5.7 months. The average LBBAP success rate was 89.6% with a success rate better for bradyarrhythmia (92.4%) as compared to HF indication (82.2%). Common reasons for implantation failure were inability to penetrate deep into the interventricular septum, septal fibrosis, inability to reach the target area due to enlarged cardiac chambers, and broad QRS morphology or nonspecific intraventricular conduction delay (NIVCD). NIVCD denotes that the patient has more of a myocardial disease than a mere electrical abnormality leading to ventricular dysfunction. Thus, LBBAP will not be sufficient to improve outcomes in these cases. Similar reasons were observed by Vijayaraman et al. group and the cases done at our center. Based on these outcomes we can choose our patients upfront for LBBAP in lieu of BiVP among the HF group as shown in **Table 1**. Complications observed during the procedure and on follow-up were acute perforation into the

TABLE 1: Case selection for LBBAP or BiVP in patients with heart failure and reduced ejection fraction (HFrEF) with wide QRS.

LBBAP	BiVP
Typical LBBB with NICMP	LBBB with ICMP with septal scar
Pacing induced CMP	NIVCD with HFrEF
Masquerading bundle branch block with NICMP	Structural heart diseases with septal scar, e.g., cardiac sarcoidosis, myocardial tuberculosis, hypertrophic cardiomyopathy, inherited cardiomyopathy

(BiVP: biventricular pacing; LBBAP: left bundle branch area pacing; NICMP: nonischemic cardiomyopathy; NIVCD: nonspecific intraventricular conduction delay)

left ventricular (LV) cavity, acute coronary syndrome, coronary vein fistula, coronary artery fistula, trapped lead/damaged helix, delayed perforation into LV cavity, rise in threshold and lead dislodgment in total 11.7% of patients. These complication rates are comparable with the BiVP complication rate. The majority of these were considered minor complications which could be managed conservatively. There were no deaths, strokes, or thromboembolic events. As per the proposed criteria, LBFP was the predominant capture type in 69.5% of patients followed by LVSP in 21.5%, and true LBBP was achieved in only 9% of patients. QRS interval was shorter for LBFP as compared to LBBP and LVSP. Despite this wide variety of LBBAP, there was no difference in the outcome among these groups over 6.4 ± 5.7 months' follow-up.

Thus, we still need better implant tools, techniques, and criteria to further improve the outcome of physiologic pacing in both bradyarrhythmia and HF indications.

Key messages

- LBBAP is feasible in both bradyarrhythmia and HF indications.
- Majority of patients achieve LBF capture or LVS capture instead of main LBB capture, with no major difference in the outcome among these groups.
- Success rate of LBBAP is better with bradyarrhythmia (92.4%) indication as compared to HF (82.2%).

ARTICLE 3

Predictors for Early Mortality in Patients with Implantable Cardiac Defibrillator for Heart Failure with Reduced Ejection Fraction

Çinier G, Hayıroğlu Mİ, Çınar T, Pay L, Yumurtaş AÇ, Tezen O, et al. Predictors for early mortality in patients with implantable cardiac defibrillator for heart failure with reduced ejection fraction.
Indian Heart J. 2022;74(2):127-30.

Abstract

In heart failure, implantable cardioverter-defibrillator (ICD) are suggested in patients suffering from heart failure with reduced ejection fraction (HFrEF) to decrease arrhythmic death rate. Present study was designed to determine risk factors associated with mortality following the ICD in 1 year. We have extracted data from our hospital's electronic database system for those patients who were implanted ICD secondary to HFrEF from the year 2009 to 2019. A total of 1,107 patients were registered in the present study. In this study, we have observed 4.7% mortality rate at 1-year following the device implantation time. On applying multivariate analysis, age, atrial fibrillation, New York Heart Association (NYHA) classification >2, blood urea nitrogen, pro-brain natriuretic peptide, and albumin independently indicated 1-year mortality.

ARTICLE COMMENTARY

In the research brief published in the Indian Heart Journal (IHJ), the authors Goksel Cinier, et al. have analyzed the first-year mortality in patients with ICD implants. Of the 1,107 patients in the study, 54 patients died. This amounts to a mortality rate of 4.7%. The authors also report predictors of mortality. Old age, diabetes mellitus, ischemic heart failure, atrial fibrillation, and higher New York Heart Association (NYHA) class were among the strong predictors of mortality. The authors also report the incidence of appropriate shocks (4.4%) and inappropriate shocks (1.2%). Among the blood markers, low albumin and high blood urea were significant predictors of mortality.

The 1-year mortality rate of 4.7%, immediately after ICD implant, reported in this study is lower compared to the annual mortality rate of around 10% reported in randomized control trials. It is possible that contemporary medical treatment has reduced the mortality rates. Nevertheless, the predictors of mortality seem to be the same as described in another similar study (the Israel ICD registry). The latter study had, in fact, proposed a score–AAACC ("triple A double C") score for prediction of 1-year mortality after ICD implantation: Age >75 years, atrial fibrillation, anemia, chronic lung disease, and chronic renal failure.

Key messages

- Presence of comorbidities like renal dysfunction, lung disease increases the risk of nonarrhythmic mortality.
- Old age is consistently a risk marker of early mortality despite ICD implant. This points to a higher incidence of nonarrhythmic deaths in the elderly. This calls for a randomized control study in the elderly patients with heart failure and reduced ejection fraction to address whether ICD intervention truly brings down the mortality rate.
- Use of artificial intelligence derived from large databases would probably help in deriving a comprehensive score model to predict mortality risk in ICD recipients. This would help us in reallocating ICD resources to the most needy patients.

ARTICLE 4

Predictors of Primary Prevention Implantable Cardioverter-defibrillator Use in Heart Failure with Reduced Ejection Fraction: Impact of the Predicted Risk of Sudden Cardiac Death and All-cause Mortality

Schrage B, Lund LH, Benson L, Dahlström U, Shadman R, Linde C, et al. Predictors of primary prevention implantable cardioverter-defibrillator use in heart failure with reduced ejection fraction: impact of the predicted risk of sudden cardiac death and all-cause mortality.
Eur J Heart Fail. 2022;24(7):1212-22.

Abstract

Aims: For primary prevention of sudden cardiac death (SCD) in heart failure with reduced ejection fraction (HFrEF), the use of implantable cardioverter-defibrillators (ICD) is limited. The present study aimed to examine barriers to ICD use in HFrEF even though considering the predicted risk of mortality and SCD.

Method and results: SwedeHF registered from the year 2011–2018 and suspected for primary prevention of ICD was analyzed. The Seattle Proportional Risk and Seattle Heart Failure Models were used to envisage the proportional SCD and all-cause mortality risk, respectively. For the identification of independent predictors of ICD use/nonuse, a multivariable logistic regression model was applied; Cox regression models were used to evaluate the interaction between predicted SCD/mortality risk and ICD use for mortality. Out of 13,475 patients, only 15.5% had the ICD. Those who showed higher predicted proportional SCD risk (>45%) had an ~80% higher possibility to have the ICD. Some additional predictors of nonuse were follow-up in primary versus specialty care are higher comorbidity burden and lower socioeconomic status. Use of ICD was associated with lower mortality only in higher predicted SCD patients and lower mortality risk (34% and 37% relative risk reduction for 3-year all-cause and cardiovascular mortality, respectively). In this subgroup of patients, 81.8% of ICD was underuse.

Conclusion: In the modern-day registry, patients with an indication for primary prevention ICD received device are 15.5%. Whereas, a high predicted proportional SCD risk was appropriately related to ICD use involving some factor, i.e., the lack of specialized follow-up, higher comorbidity burden, and lower socioeconomic status, the major unjustified impediments to implementation. Our findings recommended some important extents for improving ICD use for the primary prevention of SCD in clinical practice.

ARTICLE COMMENTARY

Guidelines formulated based on the evidence from randomized control trials and meta-analyses advocate implantable cardioverter-defibrillators (ICD) for primary prevention in heart failure with reduced ejection fraction (HFrEF) especially when left ventricular ejection fraction (LVEF) ≤35%. Benedikt Schrage et al., in the European

Heart Journal (EHJ), have presented their study on the real-world adoption of the ICD for the primary prevention of heart failure. The authors have conducted the study in two steps. First, they report the prevalence of ICD use and underuse in patients from the SwedeHF registry, who are indicated for primary prevention. Second, they report the predictors of both the use and underuse of ICD in these patients. Finally, they also report their extended observations on the incidence of mortality and the association between deaths and ICD use according to various categories of risk. The Seattle Proportional Risk Model (SPRM) was applied to estimate the sudden cardiac death (SCD) risk and Seattle Heart Failure Model (SHFM) was applied to estimate the mortality risk in these patients.

The authors report a gross underuse of ICD of only 15.5% among the 13,475 patients who had an indication for primary prevention of ICD. Among the various predictors of ICD use, ICD adoption was better when the SCD risk was high in the cohort, heart failure duration >6 months, and in a specialty follow-up. The significant predictors for the nonuse of ICD were lower socioeconomic status and higher comorbidity burden. All-cause mortality was 25.6% in this cohort. Over a median follow-up of 2 years, 3,450 (25.6%) all-cause deaths occurred. When the association between ICD use and deaths was analyzed, the authors conclude that higher all-cause deaths were observed when the calculated SCD risk was higher, and lower all-cause deaths were observed when both the calculated mortality and SCD risk were lower.

This is a novel study in trying to understand the real-world scenario of ICD use for primary prevention. According to the authors, the results of DANISH (The Danish Study to Assess the Efficacy of ICDs in Patients With Nonischemic Systolic Heart Failure on Mortality) do not seem to have affected ICD use. Rather the authors note an increase in ICD use after DANISH study. It is possible that the DANISH study gave more clarity to the clinicians that the younger nonischemic and ischemic heart failure patients are likely to benefit from ICD for SCD reduction.

Key messages

- There seems to be a significant gap in understanding the risk for SCD. Relying on LVEF as a sole risk-stratification tool may not give a correct insight into the actual SCD risk.
- The Seattle Proportional Risk Model seems to give a good assessment of risk for SCD in patients with HFrEF.
- Adoption of ICD for patients for primary prevention by clinicians seems to be better when the SCD risk is higher, irrespective of the guideline indications.
- SCD risk is high in the presence of ischemic heart disease. Applying SCD risk scoring by the Seattle Proportional Risk Model seems to predict SCD and all-cause mortality risk.
- Adoption of ICD might increase when we have reliable risk-stratification tools like cardiac MRI, irrespective of the LVEF status.

ARTICLE 5

Cardioverter-defibrillator Reduces Mortality Risk in Eligible Ischemic and Nonischemic Cardiomyopathy Patients: Sub-analysis of the Multicenter Improve SCA Study

Singh B, Hsieh YC, Liu YB, Lin KH, Joung B, Rodriguez DA, et al. Cardioverter-defibrillator reduces mortality risk in eligible ischemic and non-ischemic cardiomyopathy patients: Sub-analysis of the multi-center Improve SCA study. *Indian Heart J. 2023;75(2):115-21.*

Abstract

Background and Objectives: In regions of Asia, Latin America, Eastern Europe, the Middle East, and Africa, regardless of the burden of sudden cardiac arrest (SCA) worldwide, implantable cardioverter-defibrillators (ICDs) are underutilized. The advance SCA trial verified that primary prevention (PP) in these regions was beneficial for patients from an ICD or a cardiac resynchronization therapy with defibrillator (CRT-D). This study was planned to compare the rate of device therapy and mortality among ischemic and nonischemic cardiomyopathy (ICM and NICM) PP patients compatible for guideline indications provided for ICD therapy and had an ICD/CRT-D implanted.

Methods: In present study, patients were enrolled from the above-mentioned regions to improve SCA, nonrandomized, and nonblinded multicenter trial. Analysis of all-cause mortality and device therapy were inspected by performing cardiomyopathy (ICM vs. NICM) and implantation status. Here used Cox proportional hazards methods for adjusting factors that affect mortality risk.

Results: Out of 1,848 PP NICM patients, 1,007 (54.5%) received ICD/CRT-D, while 303 out of 581 (52.1%) PP ICM patients received an ICD/CRT-D. NICM patients at 3 years with and without an ICD/CRT-D were 13.1% and 18.3%, respectively [hazard ratio (HR) 0.51; 95% confidence interval (CI) 0.38–0.68, $p < 0.001$] for all-cause mortality rate. Likewise, all-cause mortality at 3 years in ICM patients was 13.8% in those with a device and 19.9% in those without an ICD/CRT-D (HR 0.54; 95% CI 0.33–0.88; $p = 0.011$). Here, not any significant difference between two groups was found ($p = 0.263$) at time to first device therapy, time to first shock, and time to first antitachycardia pacing (ATP) therapy.

Conclusion: Defibrillator device implantation considered as a significant benefit of mortality in both NICM and ICM patients in this present large data set of patients with a guideline-based PP ICD indication. In both groups, the rate of appropriate device therapy was similar.

ARTICLE COMMENTARY

In this subanalysis of the IMPROVE-SCA study, the authors Balbir Singh, et al. report the mortality in patients with and without implantable cardioverter-defibrillator (ICD) in both ischemic (ICM) and nonischemic cardiomyopathy (NICM). This study is one of the few studies representing population from low- and middle-income countries in Asia, South America, Eastern Europe, the Middle East, and Africa. In this cohort, there were

2,420 patients eligible for primary prevention according to guideline recommendations. However, only 54.5% of the eligible NICM received ICD and 52.1% of eligible ICM received ICD. ICD patients had a significantly lower all-cause mortality in both the NICM (3-year all-cause mortality 13.8%) and ICM groups (3-year all-cause mortality 13.1%), compared to those patients with no ICD (NICM 3-year all-cause mortality 18.3% and ICM 3-year all-cause mortality 19.9%). Compared to ICM (3-year all-cause mortality 13.1%), the mortality reduction observed was even greater in the NICM group (3-year all-cause mortality 13.8%).

While the results of this study are in line with the Sudden Cardiac Death in Heart Failure Trial (SCD-HeFT) outcomes, the results contradict the outcomes of DANISH (The Danish Study to Assess the Efficacy of ICDs in Patients With Nonischemic Systolic Heart Failure on Mortality) study. While the DANISH study was a randomized control trial in a singular population belonging to Denmark, the IMPROVE-SCA study is a real-world study representing Asia, Africa, and America. Moreover, the survival benefit seems to be similar in ICM and NICM patients receiving ICD for primary prevention.

Key messages

- The subanalysis of the IMPROVE-SCA study advocates for ICD for primary prevention in NICM and ICM patients according to guideline recommendations.
- Though the study is not a randomized control study, the results are more representative of a wider geographical region.

ARTICLE 6

Rivaroxaban in Rheumatic Heart Disease-associated Atrial Fibrillation

Connolly SJ, Karthikeyan G, Ntsekhe M, Haileamlak A, El Sayed A, El Ghamrawy A, et al. Rivaroxaban in Rheumatic Heart Disease-Associated Atrial Fibrillation.
N Engl J Med. 2022;387(11):978-88.

Abstract

Background: Limited testing of factor Xa inhibitors has been reported till date for the prevention strategies of cardiovascular events in patients with rheumatic heart disease-associated atrial fibrillation.

Methods: Patients presented with the complaint of atrial fibrillation confirmed by echocardiographically with rheumatic heart disease (RHD) who had shown any of the described characteristics: a CHA_2DS_2-VASc score of at least 2 (on a scale from 0 to 9, with higher scores indicating a higher risk of stroke), a mitral-valve area of no >2 cm², left atrial spontaneous echo contrast, or left atrial thrombus were enrolled. For present study, patients were randomly selected to receive standard doses of rivaroxaban and dose-adjusted vitamin K antagonists (VKAs). The major efficacy outcome involves composite of stroke, systemic embolism, myocardial infarction, or death from vascular (cardiac or noncardiac) or unfamiliar causes. We assumed that rivaroxaban therapy would be noninferior to the vitamin K antagonist therapy. According to the International Society of Thrombosis and Hemostasis, the most important safety outcome was major bleeding.

Results: Of the total enrolled 4,565 patients, for final analysis 4,531 were included. The average age of the patients was observed, 50.5 years and of which 72.3% were women. More common permanent discontinuation of trial medication was seen with rivaroxaban than with vitamin K antagonist therapy at every visit. The primary-outcome events were seen in 560 patients in the rivaroxaban group and 446 in the vitamin K antagonist group, in the intention-to-treat analysis. Survival curves were observed to be nonproportional. In the rivaroxaban group noted the restricted mean survival time was 1,599 days and in the vitamin K antagonist group, 1,675 days [difference: −76 days; 95% confidence interval (CI) −121 to −31; $p < 0.001$). It was observed that there were more incidence of death occurred in the rivaroxaban group than in group of vitamin K antagonist (restricted mean survival time: 1,608 days vs. 1,680 days; difference: −72 days; 95% CI −117 to −28). For rate of major bleeding no significant difference between groups was noted.

Conclusion: Among rheumatic heart disease patients-associated with atrial fibrillation, vitamin K antagonist therapy simply directed to show a lower rate of cardiovascular events or death events than rivaroxaban therapy, without reporting a higher rate of bleeding incidences.

ARTICLE COMMENTARY

Rheumatic heart disease (RHD) affects over 40 million people, particularly in low/middle-income countries (LMICs). About 20% of symptomatic RHD patients have atrial fibrillation (AF) and vitamin K antagonists (VKAs) are the current standard of care for stroke prevention in these patients. However, less than half of these patients are actually prescribed VKA, and even when they are used, there is a tendency to under anticoagulant, as shown in the Indian Heart Rhythm Society-Atrial Fibrillation (IHRS-AF) registry in which the reported average international normalized ratios (INR) of the entire cohort over 1 year was 1.8.[1] Overall just one-third may achieve therapeutic INR.[2] Direct oral anticoagulants (DOACs) have emerged as strong contenders for stroke prevention in AF over the last decade, driven by evidence from multiple randomized controlled trials, and have established noninferiority (additional 10% mortality reduction) over VKAs in this subset.[3] The noninferiority of DOACs to VKAs has also been studied in patients with AF and bioprosthetic heart valves. *However, moderate-to-severe rheumatic mitral stenosis and mechanical heart valves are two such clinical situations where DOACs have not found data-driven clinical supremacy.* The Investigation of Rheumatic AF Treatment Using Vitamin K Antagonists, Rivaroxaban or Aspirin Studies (INVICTUS) investigators, in their randomized controlled trial, compared once-daily rivaroxaban (20 mg or 15 mg based on creatinine clearance) with dose-adjusted VKA (warfarin or acenocoumarol) in documented RHD and AF. The trial enrolled 4,565 patients with AF and echocardiographically proven RHD with one of the following: CHA_2DS_2-VASc ≥2, mitral valve area 2 cm² or echocardiographic evidence of left atrial or appendage thrombus. Main exclusion criteria were the existence of a mechanical heart valve or the likelihood of receiving one in the next 6 months among others.[4] Enrollment continued for 3 years and the average follow-up duration was 3.1 years. The event-driven primary outcome which initially comprised only stroke and systemic embolism had to be revised in the course of the study to include death from any cause (Based on the assumption that most deaths with unknown causes were vascular) because of lesser than expected strokes and an unprecedented high number of deaths. As for the results, death and stroke (especially ischemic stroke) occurred more frequently in the group of rivaroxaban than in the VKA group, and there was no substantial difference in the rate of bleeding. The striking (and rather unexpected) difference in mortality was almost wholly due to increased rates of sudden death and of death because of mechanical or pump failure in the rivaroxaban group, and there was no significant difference between-group in the rate of hospitalization for heart failure.

While the absolute difference in the number of strokes was small (25), there were 110 more deaths in the rivaroxaban group. The stroke reduction in the VKA group cannot be commented on in this underpowered study. Nevertheless, more frequent drug discontinuations in the rivaroxaban group can be postulated as contributing to this.

The striking mortality reduction in the VKA group does not sync with the results of trials in nonrheumatic AF where the benefit was driven by reduction in mortality from hemorrhagic stroke. The authors have come up with a proposition citing the potential disease-modifying effect of VKAs. However, the same was not reflected in the number of patients subjected to valve surgery which was similar in the two groups. *The only other thing that can explain the outcome difference is the frequency of in-person clinic follow-ups which were far more frequent in the VKA group because of the need for frequent INR monitoring. One has to understand that outcomes in the RHD population which is far younger than nonvalvular AF are dependent upon a holistic overall approach and not simply stroke prevention.*

The INVICTUS trial for the first ever time has brought forth the need to look beyond stroke prevention in rheumatic AF and does not completely sideline DOACs despite the contradicting results. For the time being, as per current treatment guidelines VKAs should be used for stroke prevention in patients with RHD and AF.

ARTICLE 7

Randomized Ablation-based Rhythm-control versus Rate-control Trial in Patients with Heart Failure and Atrial Fibrillation: Results from the RAFT-AF trial

Parkash R, Wells GA, Rouleau J, Talajic M, Essebag V, Skanes A, et al. Randomized Ablation-Based Rhythm-Control Versus Rate-Control Trial in Patients With Heart Failure and Atrial Fibrillation: Results from the RAFT-AF trial. *Circulation. 2022;145(23):1693-704.*

Abstract

Background: Treatment of coexisting atrial fibrillation (AF) and heart failure (HF) can be not that easy. Pharmacologically based rhythm control of AF has not been verified to be superior to rate control. On performing the comparison of ablation-based rhythm control with rate control, to assess whether clinical outcomes in patients with HF and AF could be improved or not.

Methods: Present study was a multicenter, open-label trial with blinded outcome evaluation using a central adjudication committee. Random assignment to ablation-based rhythm control or rate control in patients with high-burden paroxysmal (more than four episodes in 6 months) or persistent (duration <3 years) AF, New York Heart Association (NYHA) class II to III HF, and elevated NT-proBNP (N-terminal pro–B-type natriuretic peptide). With a minimum follow-up of 2 years, the primary endpoint decided for the study was a composite of all-cause mortality and all HF events. The secondary outcomes mainly consist of left ventricular ejection fraction, 6-minute walk test (6MWT), and NT-proBNP. Using the Minnesota Living with Heart Failure Questionnaire (MLHFQ) Quality of life (QOL) was measured. Also, AF effect was measured on QOL. Cox proportional hazards modeling was used for the primary analysis of time-to-event. Due to the determination of superficial ineffectiveness by the Data and Safety Monitoring Committee (DSMC), the trial was stopped early.

Results: A total of 411 patients were randomly assigned to ablation-based rhythm control (n = 214) or rate control (n = 197) from 1st December 2011 to 20th January 2018. The most important outcome was seen in the ablation-based rhythm control group, 50 (23.4%) patients, and in the rate-control group, 64 (32.5%) patients [hazard ratio (HR) 0.71 (95% CI 0.49–1.03); $p = 0.066$]. The observed increase in eft ventricular ejection fraction in the ablation-based group (10.1 ± 1.2% vs. 3.8 ± 1.2%, $p = 0.017$), 6MWT improved (44.9 ± 9.1 m vs. 27.5 ± 9.7 m, $p = 0.025$), and a decrease in NT-proBNP (mean change −77.1% vs. −39.2%, $p < 0.0001$). In the ablation-based rhythm-control group MLHFQ demonstrated greater improvement [least-squares mean difference of −5.4 (95% CI −10.5 to −0.3); $p = 0.0036$], as did the AF Effect on QOL score [least-squares mean difference of 6.2 (95% CI 1.7–10.7); $p = 0.0005$]. In 50% of patients in both treatment groups, serious adverse events were observed.

Conclusion: Present study concludes that there was no significant statistical difference in all-cause mortality or HF events with ablation-based rhythm control versus rate control in high-burden AF patients and HF patients; while, there was a nonsignificant trend for improved outcomes with ablation-based rhythm control over rate control.

ARTICLE COMMENTARY

The debate has always been "Rate versus Rhythm control" in atrial fibrillation (AF) and rhythm control could never reign supreme over rate control.[4] As such, rhythm control strategy has traditionally been thought to improve "Quality of Life (QOL)" with no significant mortality benefit. This is because pharmacologic strategies are often associated with drug-induced adverse events.[5] AF with heart failure (HF) is a particularly challenging subset of patients to treat as there are up to 40% higher odds of death as compared to those in sinus rhythm (SR).[6] The updated 2022 American Heart Association/American College of Cardiology/Heart Failure Society of America guidelines for the management of heart failure provide a Class IIa recommendation for catheter ablation (CA) for patients with heart failure and symptoms caused by AF "to improve symptoms and quality of life".[7] This evidence stems from the AATAC (Ablation vs. Amiodarone for Treatment of Atrial Fibrillation in Patients With Congestive Heart Failure and an Implanted ICD/CRTD; 203 patients) and CASTLE-AF (Catheter Ablation for Atrial Fibrillation With Heart Failure; 363 patients).[8,9] However, a reduction in death and hospitalization was seen in secondary outcomes in the former, and the target sample size was not reached in the latter.

The RAFT-AF (Randomized Ablation-based Rhythm-Control versus Rate-Control Trial in Patients with Heart Failure and Atrial Fibrillation) trial tried to find out if CA-based rhythm control can help to improve outcomes in patients with symptomatic HF (irrespective of ejection fraction) and elevated NT-proBNP; and high burden of paroxysmal/persistent AF. The CA group underwent pulmonary vein isolation (PVI) as default in the paroxysmal AF subset and PVI plus additional lesion sets in the persistent AF population. They were additionally treated with antiarrhythmics (amiodarone, dofetilide, and sotalol) based on the treating physician's discretion. The rate control group received β-blockers, calcium-channel blockers, and/or digoxin. Drug-refractory cases underwent atrio-ventricular nodal ablation followed by cardiac resynchronization therapy. Approximately two-thirds of the study participants ($n = 411$) had EF < 40%, the majority had persistent AF (type 2 to >7 days) and after a minimum follow-up period of 2 years, the trial showed a modest nonsignificant benefit in the primary composite outcome of all-cause mortality or HF events with ablation-based rhythm control over rate control in patients [50 out of 214 (23.4%) in the ablation-based rhythm-control group compared with 64 out of 197 (32.5%)] in the rate-control group [HR 0.71; (95% CI 0.49–1.03); $p = 0.066$]. Similar trend was noted in the prespecified subgroup analysis of patients with EF < 45%. Secondary outcomes of 6-minute walk test, change in EF, NT-proBNP all favored CA.

The results of this underpowered study (with an original sample size of 1,000 and subsequent planned size of 400) should be interpreted with the knowledge that the outcomes could have reached significance had the "Data Monitoring" committee not recommended stopping the trial prematurely for futility at the interim analysis. The reasons for such a recommendation were slower recruitment and a trend for worse outcomes with CA till that time. However, the final results showed a trend toward the opposite. *Hence, this could be seen as a missed opportunity and serve as a lesson to the fact that interim analysis can be unreliable as trials are generally executed for the planned sample size and follow-up.* Landmark trials like ISIS-2 (Second International Study of Infarct Survival) were allowed to continue despite the risk of futility in the interim analysis. Moreover, CA techniques have greatly evolved over the last decade with better outcomes.

Reviewing all the facts, it can be inferred that if the RAFT-AF trial had been carried to completion, the results may have been much more valuable. Nevertheless, it adds to the literature suggesting the benefit of CA for HF with reduced EF. Additional adequately powered trials are required to assess if CA-based rhythm control strategies for AF and heart failure could reduce mortality and heart failure events.

REFERENCES

1. Watkins DA, Johnson CO, Colquhoun SM, Karthikeyan G, Beaton A, Bukhman G, et al. Global, regional, and national burden of rheumatic heart disease, 1990-2015. N Engl J Med. 2017;377(8):713-22.
2. Ruff CT, Giugliano RP, Braunwald E, Hoffman EB, Deenadayalu N, Ezekowitz MD, et al. Comparison of the efficacy and safety of new oral anticoagulants with warfarin in patients with atrial fibrillation: a meta-analysis of randomised trials. Lancet. 2014; 383:955-62.
3. Connolly SJ, Karthikeyan G, Ntsekhe M, Haileamlak A, El Sayed A, El Ghamrawy A, et al. Rivaroxaban in rheumatic heart disease-associated atrial fibrillation. N Engl J Med. 2022;387:978-88.
3. Hindricks G, Potpara T, Dagres N, Arbelo E, Bax JJ, Blomström-Lundqvist C, et al. 2020 ESC Guidelines for the diagnosis and management of atrial fibrillation developed in collaboration with the European Association for Cardio-Thoracic Surgery (EACTS): the task force for the diagnosis and management of atrial fibrillation of the European Society of Cardiology (ESC) developed with the special contribution of the European Heart Rhythm Association (EHRA) of the ESC. Eur Heart J. 2021;42:373-498.
4. Sethi NJ, Feinberg J, Nielsen EE, Safi S, Gluud C, Jakobsen JC. The effects of rhythm control strategies versus rate control strategies for atrial fibrillation and atrial flutter: A systematic review with meta-analysis and Trial Sequential Analysis. PLoS One. 2017;12(10):e0186856.
5. January CT, Wann LS, Calkins H, Chen LY, Cigarroa JE, Cleveland JC Jr, et al. 2019 AHA/ACC/HRS focused update of the 2014 AHA/ACC/HRS guideline for the manage- ment of patients with atrial fibrillation: a report of the American College of Cardiology/American Heart Association Task Force on Clinical Practice Guidelines and the Heart Rhythm Society. Circulation. 2019;140:e125-51.
6. Mamas MA, Caldwell JC, Chacko S, Garratt CJ, Fath-Ordoubadi F, Neyses L. A meta-analysis of the prognostic significance of atrial fibrillation in chronic heart failure. Eur J Heart Fail. 2009;11:676-83.
7. Heidenreich PA, Bozkurt B, Aguilar D, Allen LA, Byun JJ, Colvin MM, et al. 2022 AHA/ACC/ HFSA guideline for the management of heart failure: a report of the American College of Cardiology/American Heart Association Joint Committee on Clinical Practice Guidelines. Circulation. 2022;145:e895-1032.
8. Di Biase L, Mohanty P, Mohanty S, Santangeli P, Trivedi C, Lakkireddy D, et al. Ablation versus amiodarone for treatment of persistent atrial fibrillation in patients with congestive heart failure and an implanted device: results from the AATAC multicenter randomized trial. Circulation. 2016;133:1637-44.
9. Marrouche NF, Kheirkhahan M, Brachmann J. Catheter ablation for atrial fibrillation with heart failure. N Engl J Med. 2018;379:492.

SECTION 8
Heart Failure in Women

Section Editor: **Justin Paul**

Co-Editor: Arpita Katheria

ARTICLE 1

Infertility and Risk of Heart Failure in the Women's Health Initiative

Lau ES, Wang D, Roberts M, Taylor CN, Murugappan G, Shadyab AH, et al. Infertility and Risk of Heart Failure in the Women's Health Initiative.
J Am Coll Cardiol. 2022;79(16):1594-603.

Abstract

Background: Previous known information indicated that there is an association of reproductive factors with an increased risk of future cardiovascular (CV) disease. However, emerging data support its association with increased risk of CV disease and infertility but not enough is well-known about the same. The association of infertility with future risk of heart failure (HF) is not fully understood and is presently the current research interest topic.

Objectives: In women with and without a history of infertility present study aimed to examine the development of HF and HF subtypes.

Methods: Postmenopausal women were followed by the Women's Health Initiative prospectively for the development of HF. At the study baseline, infertility was self-reported. To evaluate the association of infertility with incident overall HF and HF subtypes [heart failure with preserved ejection fraction (HFpEF): left ventricular ejection fraction of ≥50% vs. heart failure with reduced ejection fraction (HFrEF): left ventricular ejection fraction of <50%] multivariable cause-specific Cox models were used.

Results: Among 38,528 postmenopausal women (mean age: 63 ± 7 years), a history of infertility was reported by 5,399 (14%) participants. A total of 2,373 participants developed HF incidents, including 807 with HFrEF and 1,133 with HFpEF over a median follow-up of 15 years. Also, observed that there was an independent association of infertility with future risk of overall HF (HR 1.16; 95% CI 1.04–1.30; $p = 0.006$). Remarkably, on examining subtypes of HF, infertility was found to be associated with future risk of HFpEF (HR 1.27; 95% CI 1.09–1.48; $p = 0.002$) but not with HFrEF (HR 0.97; 95% CI 0.80–1.18).

> **Conclusion:** Infertility was significantly associated with incident HF. This was driven by an increased risk of HFpEF, but not HFrEF, and appeared independent of traditional CV risk factors and other infertility-related conditions. Future research should investigate mechanisms that underlie the link between infertility and HFpEF.

ARTICLE COMMENTARY

This study examines the association of infertility with the risk of heart failure (HF) and HF subtypes among women enrolled in the Women's Health Initiative (WHI). WHI is a national prospective study of 161,808 postmenopausal women recruited across 40 clinical centers between 1993 and 1998. The present study analyzed 38,528 postmenopausal women with centrally adjudicated HF outcomes from the HF subcohort of WHI. Infertility was self-reported at the study baseline. Multivariable cause-specific Cox models were used to evaluate the association of infertility with incident overall HF and HF subtypes [heart failure with preserved ejection fraction (HFpEF) vs. heart failure with reduced ejection fraction (HFrEF)]. The association of infertility with established congenital heart defect (CHD) risk factors [age, body mass index (BMI), race/ethnicity, systolic blood pressure, hypertension treatment, diabetes mellitus (DM), smoking status, and hyperlipidemia] was also evaluated. The association of infertility-related risk factors (irregular menses, thyroid disease, waist circumference, and early menopause) with HF was analyzed.

About 5,399 (14%) of the 38,528 postmenopausal women reported a history of infertility. Over a median follow-up time of 15 years [interquartile range (IQR) 8–20], 2,373 women developed incident HF, including 807 HFrEF cases and 1,133 HFpEF cases. Infertility was independently associated with future risk of HF. Women with infertility had a nearly 20% increased risk of developing HF compared with those without infertility. This association was primarily for HFpEF (HR 1.27; $p < 0.002$) but not HFrEF (HR 0.97). Infertility was not associated with 10-year atherosclerotic cardiovascular disease (ASCVD) risk.

The statistical model demonstrated significant associations between irregular menses, early menopause, and thyroid disease with infertility. Thyroid disease and early menopause were also associated with future risk of overall HF (HR 1.11). The relationship between infertility and future risk of HF and HFpEF persisted even after further adjustment for irregular menses, early menopause, and thyroid disease.

Women with infertility had a higher risk of developing HF. This was driven primarily by an increased risk of future HFpEF, but not HFrEF.

The increased risk of HF in women with a history of infertility was not explained by traditional atherosclerotic cardiovascular (CV) risk factors such as hypertension, obesity, and DM or a greater risk of ischemic heart disease. This increased risk was not also explained by the risk factors for infertility like menstrual cycle irregularity, premature menopause, and hypothyroidism.

Taken together, these findings support the novel association of infertility with incident HFpEF, which appears independent of traditional CV risk factors, ischemic heart disease, or infertility-associated factors. The findings suggest that the mechanisms mediating HF risk in infertility are orthogonal to traditional ASCVD. Future research should investigate mechanisms that underlie the link between infertility and HFpEF. A potential limitation of the study is the reliance on self-reported infertility status, which introduces the possibility of misclassification.

Key messages

- A woman's reproductive period is becoming an increasingly important window into her lifetime CV risk. Premature menopause and adverse pregnancy outcomes, including hypertensive disorders of pregnancy and gestational diabetes, are well-recognized as independent risk factors for future ASCVD.
- This study has presented evidence supporting infertility as an independent risk factor for the development of HF among women without previous history of HF.

ARTICLE 2

Distinct Pathophysiological Pathways in Women and Men with Heart Failure

Ravera A, Santema BT, de Boer RA, Anker SD, Samani NJ, Lang CC, et al. Distinct Pathophysiological Pathways in Women and Men with Heart Failure.
Eur J Heart Fail. 2022;24(9):1532-44.

Abstract

Aims: In heart failure (HF), the clinical differences between women and men have been described widely. Still, limited knowledge is known about the underlying pathophysiological mechanisms. Hence, in this present study, comparisons of multiple circulating biomarkers were planned to gain better insights into differential HF pathophysiology between women and men.

Methods and results: Compared differential expression of a panel of 363 biomarkers in 537 women and 1,485 men with HF. To identify differential biological pathways in women and men, performed a pathway overrepresentation analysis. In an independent HF cohort (575 women and 1,123 men) all findings were validated. Women were older and had higher left ventricular ejection fraction (LVEF) observed in both cohorts. Found 14/363 and 12/363 biomarkers that were relatively upregulated in women, while 21/363 and 14/363 were upregulated in men in the index and validation cohorts, respectively. Leptin and fatty acid binding protein-4 were the strongest upregulated biomarkers in women in both cohorts, compared to matrix metalloproteinase-3 in men. In a subset of patients from both cohorts matched by age and LVEF similar findings were pretended. In women, pathway overrepresentation analysis showed increased activity of pathways associated with lipid metabolism and in men neuroinflammatory response (all $p < 0.0001$).

Conclusion: Biomarkers associated with lipid metabolic pathways were detected in women, while biomarkers associated with neuroinflammatory response were more active in men in two independent cohorts of HF patients. In clinical phenotype observed in HF patients, differences in inflammatory and metabolic pathways may contribute to sex differences and give useful insights toward the development of personalized HF therapies.

ARTICLE COMMENTARY

Clinical differences between women and men have been well defined in heart failure (HF). Though, the gender differences in the underlying pathophysiological mechanisms have not been well elucidated. The authors ventured to understand the sex differences in pathophysiological pathways of heart failure by comparing differential expression of circulating biomarkers in men and women.

The BIOSTAT-CHF (Systems Biology Study to Tailored Treatment in Chronic Heart Failure) was a European project. This project includes two prospective, observational, multinational cohorts. To inspect the biomarker profiles in both BIOSTAT-CHF indices, about 363 distinctive proteins from different pathophysiological domains were used and validated in the present planned cohorts.

The index cohort consisted of 2,516 patients with signs and symptoms of deteriorating HF and either a left ventricular ejection fraction (LVEF) ≤ 40%, or plasma concentrations of N-terminal pro-B-type natriuretic peptide (NT-proBNP) > 2,000 ng/L, from 11 centers in Europe of the BIOSTAT-CHF project. At the time of enrollment, these patients were either receiving <50% of the target dose of angiotensin-converting enzyme inhibitors (ACEIs)/angiotensin receptor blockers (ARBs) or treatment naïve and were receiving β-blockers.

The validation cohort consisted of 1,738 patients from a second independent cohort from six centers in Scotland, with HF and a previous documented HF admission requiring diuretic treatment, not previously treated or receiving ≤50% of target doses of ACEI/ARBs and/or β-blockers.

In the present cohort, it was observed that as compared to men 14 biomarkers were found to be upregulated in women, and in the other hand, compared to women in men a total of 21 biomarkers were found to be upregulated. Leptin and fatty-acid binding protein-4 (FABP-4) was the most prominently upregulated biomarkers in women as compared with men. Matrix metalloproteinase-3 (MMP-3) was found to be the most significantly upregulated biomarker in men as compared with women. Similar findings were obtained in the validation cohort too.

Four pathways that were specifically enhanced in women with HF revealed by pathway overrepresentation analysis of the 14 upregulated biomarkers in women in the index cohort: (1) triglyceride catabolic process, (2) glycerolipid catabolic process, (3) plasma lipoprotein assembly, remodeling, and clearance, and (4) cellular response to low-density lipoprotein (LDL) particle stimulus. Similar findings were observed in the validation cohort too.

In men in the index cohort exposed, two overexpressed pathways in men, revealed by pathway overrepresentation analysis of the 21 upregulated biomarkers these are: (1) neuroinflammatory response and (2) regulation of neuroinflammatory response.

However, in the validation cohort, the upregulated biomarkers in men were less and not that enough to yield results from pathway overrepresentation analysis.

With all-cause mortality, most of the differentially expressed biomarkers showed a significant association on performing regression analysis, before and after adjustment for selected covariates.

Out of the 363 biomarkers that were evaluated 14 and 12 were relatively upregulated in women in the index and validation cohorts respectively, while 21 and 14 were upregulated in men.

Most of the differentially expressed biomarkers were significantly associated with all-cause mortality, after adjustment for selected covariates. Growth hormone-1, FABP4, and as compared to women myoglobin revealed a stronger association with adverse prognosis in men.

In women observed that some biomarkers are associated with lipid metabolic pathways were more active, although biomarkers associated with neuroinflammatory response were found to be more active in men. This could contribute to the observed differences in the clinical phenotype of HF.

Key messages

- There are sex differences in the expression of biomarkers involved in heart failure pathophysiology.
- This study has the potential to trigger more research in the field of heart failure by harnessing the possible differences in pathophysiology in men and women.

ARTICLE 3

Heart Failure Subtypes and Cardiomyopathies in Women

DeFilippis EM, Beale A, Martyn T, Agarwal A, Elkayam U, Lam CSP, et al. Heart Failure Subtypes and Cardiomyopathies in Women.
Circ Res. 2022;130(4):436-54.

Abstract

In the United States, heart failure affects over 2.6 million women and 3.4 million men with known sex differences in epidemiology, management, and response to treatment. The outcomes across a varied spectrum of cardiomyopathies mainly contain peripartum cardiomyopathy, hypertrophic cardiomyopathy, stress cardiomyopathy, cardiac amyloidosis, and sarcoidosis. Among, these determined sex-specific considerations by the cellular effects of sex hormones on the renin–angiotensin–aldosterone system, endothelial response to injury, vascular aging, and left ventricular remodeling. In clinical trials, other sex differences are sustained by inferred bias leading to undertreatment and underrepresentation. Examining systematically the published literature over the last decade is the main aim of this narrative review.

ARTICLE COMMENTARY

Objective: Present study was designed to find out the sex differences in respect with factors like pathophysiology, epidemiology, treatment, and prognosis in heart failure (HF).

Methods: The article discusses the reported sex differences in the literature in heart failure with reduced ejection fraction (HFrEF), heart failure with preserved ejection fraction (HFrEF), and specific cardiomyopathies.

HFrEF: Women are more expected to experience nonischemic cardiomyopathy in comparison to men who are more likely to have an ischemic cardiomyopathy. Among hospitalized duration of HFrEF patients, it was observed that women when compared with men are more likely to have hypertension.

Data on sex differences in response to given therapy are frequently seen in retrospective or post hoc subgroup analyses of landmark, HF clinical trials, where data of women were not well defined and widely represented. There are the suggestions that not every HF medications benefits men and women similarly. In HF medical therapies, mostly sex hormones play an important role for some of these observed differences. It was observed that plasma renin levels are lesser in women compared with men. Furthermore, angiotensin-converting enzyme (ACE) activity, vascular response to angiotensin II, and aldosterone secretion are decreased by estrogen and increased by androgen levels. In addition, the upregulation of the angiotensin type II receptors with response to injury is significantly higher in women compared to men.

Meta-analysis of ACE inhibitors (ACEIs) trials has suggested that these drugs may not benefit women. For example, in the DIG trial, women had a higher risk of mortality without a reduction in HF hospitalizations. Women had higher serum digoxin levels despite similar doses. Newer therapies like ivabradine and sodium-glucose cotransporter-2 inhibitors (SGLT-2Is) have limited sex-specific data. The SHIFT, DAPA-HF and EMPEROR-Reduced studies have shown some benefit in spite of the underrepresentation of women in HFrEF trials.

The landmark primary prevention of implantable cardiac defibrillator (ICD) trials included few women and the meta-analysis of these trials (DEFINITE, SCD-HeFT, DINAMIT, MUSTT, and MADIT-II) showed no survival benefit for women.[1-8] Women compared to men were less likely to receive ICDs or mechanical cardiac support when indicated.

HFpEF: The prevalence of HFpEF was higher in women. AF is associated with higher morbidity and mortality in women compared with men. At all levels of CHADS-VASc score it was noted that women were less expected to take anticoagulation with direct oral anticoagulants (DOACs) for atrial fibrillation (AF) than men.

The leading cause of HF in pregnancy is peripartum cardiomyopathy (PPCM) and a crucial nonobstetric cause of maternal mortality. Successive pregnancy in women with a history of PPCM can be a big factor for relapse, particularly in those with non-recovered left ventricular (LV) systolic function. ICD, cardiac resynchronization therapy (CRT), mechanical cardiac support, and cardiac transplantation should be offered to those beyond the usual window for recovery of LV function.

ARTICLE 4

Pregnancy Outcomes in Women with Heart Disease: The Madras Medical College Pregnancy and Cardiac (M-PAC) Registry from India

Justin Paul G, Anne Princy S, Anju S, Anita S, Mary MC, Gnanavelu G, et al. Pregnancy Outcomes in Women with Heart Disease: The Madras Medical College Pregnancy and Cardiac (M-PAC) Registry from India. *Eur Heart J. 2023;44(17):1530-40.*

Abstract

Aims: The present study planned to assess the fetomaternal outcome, identify the adverse outcome predictors and test the applicability of modified WHO (mWHO) classification in pregnant women with heart disease (PWWHD) from Tamil Nadu, India.

Methods and results: In the Madras Medical College Pregnancy and Cardiac (M-PAC) Registry, 1,154 pregnant women (mean age: 26.04 ± 4.2 years) with 1,029 consecutive pregnancies were prospectively enrolled from July 2016 to December 2019. For the first time during pregnancy, the majority of women (60.5%; 623/1,029) were diagnosed with heart disease (HD). The most common was rheumatic HD (42%; 433/1,029). One-third (34.2%; 352/1,029) presented with pulmonary hypertension (PH). The primary outcomes were maternal mortality and composite maternal cardiac events (MCEs). Secondary outcomes involve fetal loss and composite adverse fetal events (AFEs). In 15.2% (156/1,029; 95% CI 13.0–17.5) pregnancies MCEs occurred. Heart failure was the most common MCE (66.0%; 103/156; 95% CI 58.0–73.4). Maternal mortality was observed to be 1.9% (20/1,029; 95% CI 1.1–2.8) with the highest rates in patients with prosthetic heart valves (PHVs) (8.6%; 6/70). Independent predictors of MCE were left ventricular systolic dysfunction (LVSD), PHVs, severe mitral stenosis, PH, and current pregnancy diagnosis of HD. The c-statistic of mWHO classification for predicting MCE and maternal death were 0.794 (95% CI 0.763–0.826) and 0.796 (95% CI 0.732–0.860). 91.2% (938/1,029; 95% CI 89.392.8) of pregnancies resulted in live births. 33.7% (347/1,029; 95% CI 30.8–36.7) of pregnancies reported AFEs.

Conclusion: In PWWHD from India, high maternal mortality was observed. In women with PHVs, PH, and LVSD highest death rates occurred. In India, the mWHO classification for risk stratification may necessitate further adaptation and validation.

ARTICLE COMMENTARY

About 1–4% of all pregnancies are burdened by heart diseases, and the numbers are on the rise in the last few decades. Maternal predisposing factors include advanced age, poor lifestyle, and better survival in women with heart diseases to reach child-bearing age. Heart disease in pregnancy not only increases morbidity and mortality in pregnant women with heart disease (PWWHD), but also is associated with worse outcomes in fetus, including abortion, stillbirth, low birth weight (LBW), and preterm delivery.

This study assesses the fetomaternal outcomes in PWWHD and tests whether the modified WHO (mWHO) classification is applicable in this patient population.

The study was a prospective observational registry conducted at Madras Medical College, from July 2016 to December 2019. They included all pregnant women during the antenatal and 1-week postpartum period [6 months in peripartum cardiomyopathy (PPCM)] and have established or newly diagnosed structural heart disease, pulmonary vascular disease, aortic disease, or rhythm disturbances (sustained symptomatic tachy- or bradyarrhythmia needing treatment before pregnancy). All enrolled patients filled out detailed questionnaire, and underwent clinical examinations, ECG, and echocardiography, categorized as per Modified WHO (mWHO) classification, and followed up during pregnancy and 1-week postpartum, with routine cardiac and obstetric care.

Out of 152,415 registered pregnancies, 1,029 PWWHD were included. Mean age was 26.04 ± 4.2 years and 86% were ≤30 years. 60.5% were diagnosed with heart disease for the first time during the current pregnancy. 66.4% of patients had acquired heart disease, of which rheumatic heart disease (RHD) was the most common (42.1%) followed by mitral valve prolapse (MVP), cardiomyopathies, arrhythmias, and PPH. 30.5% had acyanotic congenital heart disease (CHD) and 3.1% had cyanotic CHD. 91.4% of patients were in the New York Heart Association (NYHA) I–II classes. High-risk mWHO (II–III, III, and IV) categories were present in 63.8% of pregnancies. One-third of patients had pulmonary hypertension and 20% had undergone intervention or surgery prior to conception. 39% were delivered by lower segment cesarean section (LSCS), remaining were vaginal deliveries.

Maternal cardiac events (MCEs) were observed in 15.2% (the most common heart failure followed by thromboembolic events, arrhythmias, bleeding, and infective endocarditis) with maternal mortality was seen in 20 (1.9%), of which 6 had prosthetic heart valves, 5 had heart failure with reduced ejection fraction (HFrEF), 3 each had severe pulmonary hypertension (PH) and infective endocarditis (IE), and 2 had severe multiple sclerosis (MS). In multivariable analysis, prosthetic valve, left ventricular (LV) dysfunction, and pulmonary hypertension predicted MCEs and maternal deaths. Severe MS predicted MCEs but not maternal mortality.

Adverse fetal events (AFEs) occurred in 33.7% and fetal loss in 8.8% of pregnancies [abortion/medical termination of pregnancy (MTP) in 7% and intrauterine fetal demise (IUFD)/stillbirth in 1.9%]. Univariable predictors of AFEs and fetal loss were current pregnancy diagnosis, NYHA class III–IV, mWHO > II, PH, significant MS [mitral valve area (MVA) ≤1.5 cm^2], prior cardiac procedures, and drug use and cyanosis. In multivariable analysis, prosthetic heart valve, severe MS, and maternal cyanosis predicted AFEs and fetal loss while PH only predicted AFEs and not fetal loss.

The mWHO score predicted MCEs and maternal mortality with moderate discriminative power and AFEs and fetal loss with low discriminative power.

■ CONCLUSION

Pregnancy in patients with heart disease is associated with high morbidity and mortality. The mWHO classification needs to be adapted for India.

Key messages

- Pregnant patients with heart disease are at high risk for MCEs and maternal mortality, particularly those with prosthetic valves, LV dysfunction, severe MS, significant PH, NYHA class > II, and first diagnosis of heart disease during pregnancy.
- Majority of women were diagnosed for the first time with cardiac disease during pregnancy. Preconception counseling in females planning pregnancy and better screening for heart disease in the antenatal period may help in improving maternal and fetal outcomes.

ARTICLE 5

Focused Cardiac Ultrasound to Guide the Diagnosis of Heart Failure in Pregnant Women in India

Alsharqi M, Ismavel VA, Arnold L, Choudhury SS, Solomi V C, Rao S, et al. Focused Cardiac Ultrasound to Guide the Diagnosis of Heart Failure in Pregnant Women in India.
J Am Soc Echocardiogr. 2022;35(12):1281-94.

Abstract

Background: The leading causes of maternal death are cardiac complications. For prompt diagnosis cardiac imaging with echocardiography is important, but in many low-resource settings, it is not available. The aim of this current study was to identify cardiac abnormalities in pregnant women in low-resource settings and the role of focused cardiac ultrasound performed by trained obstetricians and interpreted remotely by experts.

Methods: Among 301 pregnant and postpartum women recruited from 10 hospitals a cross-sectional study was conducted across three states in India. About 22 obstetricians were trained in image acquisition using a portable cardiac ultrasound device following a simplified protocol adapted from focus-assessed transthoracic echocardiography (TTE) protocol. It involved parasternal long-axis, parasternal short-axis, and apical four-chamber views on two-dimensional and color Doppler. In the United Kingdom and India, using a standard semiquantitative assessment protocol two exerts performed independent image interpretation. Using Cohen's κ interrater agreement between the experts was examined. In women available with both focused and conventional scans diagnostic accuracy of the method was examined.

Results: Using the focused method cardiac abnormalities were identified, including valvular abnormalities (27%), rheumatic heart disease (6.6%), derangements in left ventricular size (4.7%), and function (22%), atrial dilatation (19.5%), and pericardial effusion (30%). Between the two experts, there was substantial agreement on the cardiac parameters, ranging from 93.6% (κ = 0.84) for left ventricular ejection fraction to 100% (κ = 1) for valvular disease. In 79% of the parasternal long-axis, 77% of the parasternal short-axis, and 64% of apical four-chamber views image quality was rated good. For the image quality parameters, the chance-corrected κ coefficients showed fair to moderate agreement (κ = 0.28–0.51). Compared to 36 participants there was good agreement on diagnosis between the focused method and standard echocardiography (78% agreement).

Conclusion: The simplified focused method could be used for screening cardiac problems in obstetric settings and in pregnant women can accurately identify cardiac abnormalities.

ARTICLE COMMENTARY

The estimated incidence of heart failure is 2 per 1,000 hospital births in pregnant and postpartum women in India, with a case fatality rate (CFR) of 40%. However, there is a dearth of cardiologists and echocardiography facilities in low-resource settings. Focused cardiac ultrasound (FoCUS) is performed by nonexpert healthcare providers using portable devices, and images so obtained can be interpreted by experts remotely.

In this study, authors have evaluated whether FoCUS done by trained obstetricians and interpreted remotely by experts can identify heart disease in pregnant and postpartum women in low-resource settings in India, and to study the reliability of interpretation by assessing agreement between two experts remotely reading the images independently.

It is a cross-sectional study done at 10 hospitals in India between 2019 and 2021. Subjects included pregnant or postpartum (≤12 months) females with suspected heart failure [respiratory rate ≥15 breaths/min with or without ≥1 of—raised jugular venous pressure (JVP), murmur, gallop rhythm, or lung-crackles/pink-frothy sputum]. The control group had pregnant/postpartum women (≤2 days) without heart failure. Obstetricians were trained to perform FoCUS study independently. Three echo views were obtained—PLAX, PSAX (papillary muscle), and apical 4 chamber, along with color flow Doppler at mitral, tricuspid, and aortic valves. The images were assessed for pericardial effusion, valve abnormalities, chamber enlargement, ventricular dysfunction, and thrombus by two experts remotely.

A total number of 302 patients were recruited, 116 pregnant and 180 postpartum. 172 patients were in the study group and 129 in the control group. Images of 109 participants were interpreted by two experts and standard transthoracic echocardiography (TTE) was done in 36 participants. The mean age was 25.4 years in cases and 23.7 years in controls. 54.1% of cases and 69.8% of controls were primiparous. 32.5% of cases and 2.3% of controls had hypertensive disorder. Among the cases, 58.6% had NYHA class IV symptoms, 33.6% were NYHA II–III and the remaining NYHA I. Heart failure onset was in the postpartum period in 30%, while two-thirds presented with heart failure in the antenatal period, and only 1.8% during labor. 10 patients died during the study.

Around 181 subjects were identified to have cardiac abnormality (60% of cases and 33% of controls), 154 of whom had significant disease, requiring treatment and follow-up. Among valvular pathologies, mitral valve disease (81 patients) was the most common [64 had mitral regurgitation (MR) and 17 had multiple sclerosis (MS), only 20 were diagnosed as rheumatic heart disease (RHD)]. 59 participants had tricuspid regurgitation (TR), 2 tricuspid stenosis (TS), 1 aortic stenosis (AS), and 15 had AR. 65 participants had decreased LVEF [40 had ejection fraction (EF) below 45% and the rest

45–54%]. One or more chamber enlargement was present in 118 patients, most commonly left atrium (LA) (57), followed by right atrium (RA) (28), right ventricle (RV) (19), and left ventricle (LV) (14). Regional wall motion abnormalities (RWMA) in RV was seen in six cases. Pericardial effusion was present in 89 (30%) and thrombus in four participants.

Image quality was acceptable in 92.4%, good quality images were obtained more in PLAX view (79%), followed by PSAX (75%) and A4C views (62%). Agreement between both reviewers was >90% for most parameters and agreement between FoCUS and TTE was 78%, the difference attributable to the difference in LVEF.

The focused method by obstetricians was able to identify cardiac abnormalities in pregnant women with good accuracy. This study has showed that FoCUS examination protocols and method can be adapted to use in obstetric settings to accurately identify cardiac abnormalities in pregnant women in low-resource settings.

Key messages

- *Trained obstetricians in India were able to acquire high-quality cardiac images using portable cardiac ultrasound devices following a simple protocol, which were interpreted remotely by experts following an image interpretation protocol.*
- *Extension of this type of focused cardiac ultrasound in obstetric settings, for early identification of hitherto unidentified cardiac ailments in pregnancy, is a potential implication of this study.*

REFERENCES

1. McMurray JJV, Solomon SD, Inzucchi SE, Køber L, Kosiborod MN, Martinez FA, et al; DAPA-HF Trial Committees and Investigators. Dapagliflozin in patients with heart failure and reduced ejection fraction. N Engl J Med. 2019;381:1995-2008.
2. Swedberg K, Komajda M, Böhm M, Borer JS, Ford I, Dubost-Brama A, et al.; SHIFT Investigators. Ivabradine and outcomes in chronic heart failure (SHIFT): a randomised placebo-controlled study. Lancet. 2010;376:875-85.
3. Kadish A, Dyer A, Daubert JP, Quigg R, Estes NA, Anderson KP, et al.; Defibrillators in Non-Ischemic Cardiomyopathy Treatment Evaluation (DEFINITE) Investigators. Prophylactic defibrillator implantation in patients with nonischemic dilated cardiomyopathy. N Engl J Med. 2004;350(21):2151-8.
4. Bardy GH, Lee KL, Mark DB, Poole JE, Packer DL, Boineau R, et al.; Sudden Cardiac Death in Heart Failure Trial (SCD-HeFT) Investigators. Amiodarone or an implantable cardioverter-defibrillator for congestive heart failure. N Engl J Med. 2005;352(3):225-37.
5. Mark DB, Nelson CL, Anstrom KJ, Al-Khatib SM, Tsiatis AA, Cowper PA, et al.; SCD-HeFT Investigators. Cost-effectiveness of defibrillator therapy or amiodarone in chronic stable heart failure: results from the Sudden Cardiac Death in Heart Failure Trial (SCD-HeFT). Circulation. 2006;114(2):135-42.
6. Hohnloser SH, Kuck KH, Dorian P, Roberts RS, Hampton JR, Hatala R, et al.; DINAMIT Investigators. Prophylactic use of an implantable cardioverter-defibrillator after acute myocardial infarction. N Engl J Med. 2004;351(24):2481-8.
7. Noyes K, Corona E, Zwanziger J, Hall WJ, Zhao H, Wang H, et al.; Multicenter Automatic Defibrillator Implantation Trial II. Health-related quality of life consequences of implantable cardioverter/defibrillators: results from MADIT II. Med Care. 2007;45(5)377-85.
8. Zwanziger J, Hall WJ, Dick AW, Zhao H, Mushlin AI, Hahn RM, et al. The cost effectiveness of implantable cardioverter-defibrillators: results from the Multicenter Automatic Defibrillator Implantation Trial (MADIT)–II. J Am Coll Cardiol. 2006;47(11)2310-8.

SECTION 9

Advance Therapy in the Management of Heart Failure

Section Editor: **R Ravi Kumar**

Co-Editors: Surendra Deora, Kavita Tyagi

ARTICLE 1

Five-year Outcomes in Patients with Fully Magnetically Levitated versus Axial-flow Left Ventricular Assist Devices in the MOMENTUM 3 Randomized Trial

Mehra MR, Goldstein DJ, Cleveland JC, Cowger JA, Hall S, Salerno CT, et al. Five-Year Outcomes in Patients With Fully Magnetically Levitated vs Axial-Flow Left Ventricular Assist Devices in the MOMENTUM-3 Randomized Trial. JAMA. 2022;328(12):1233-42.

Abstract

Importance: For patients with advanced heart failure, durable left ventricular assist device (LVAD) therapy has appeared as a central treatment option but is still refractory to pharmacological support; outcomes, including survival, beyond 2 years were poorly characterized.

Objective: To report the composite endpoint of survival to transplant, recovery, or LVAD support free of debilitating stroke (Modified Rankin Scale score >3) or reoperation to replace the pump 5 years after the implant in participants who received the fully magnetically levitated centrifugal-flow HeartMate-3 or axial-flow HeartMate-2 LVAD in the MOMENTUM-3 randomized trial and these were still receiving LVAD therapy at the 2-year follow-up.

Design, setting, and participants: This observational study was conducted in 69 US centers, it revealed the superiority of the centrifugal-flow LVAD to the axial-flow pump with respect to survival to transplant recovery, or LVAD support free of debilitating stroke or reoperation to replace the pump at 2 years. This is a 5-year follow-up of the MOMENTUM-3 trial. A total of 295 patients were registered from June 2019 to April 2021. The extended-phase study with a 5-year follow-up in September 2021 was completed.

Exposures: In the investigational device exemption per-protocol population, out of selected 1,020 patients, at 2 years LVAD support was still received by 536, of whom 289 the centrifugal-flow pump received by 289 and the axial-flow pump received by 247.

Main outcomes and measures: At 5 years in the per-protocol population evaluated 10 end-points, between the two groups these contain a composite of survival to transplant, recovery, or LVAD support free of debilitating stroke or reoperation to replace the pump between the centrifugal-flow and axial-flow pump groups and overall survival.

Results: Overall, 477 patients (295 registered and 182 provided limited data) of 536 patients at 2 years still receiving LVAD support contributed to the extended-phase analysis [median age, 62 years; 86 (18%) women]. The Kaplan–Meier estimate for 5 years, of survival to transplant, recovery, or LVAD support free of debilitating stroke, or reoperation to replace the pump in the centrifugal-flow versus axial-flow group was 54.0% versus 29.7% [HR 0.55 (95% CI 0.45–0.67); $p < 0.001$]. In the centrifugal-flow group, Kaplan–Meier survival was 58.4% versus in the axial-flow group 43.7% [HR 0.72 (95% CI 0.58–0.89); $p = 0.003$]. In the centrifugal-flow pump group, less frequent serious adverse events of stroke, bleeding, and pump thrombosis were noted.

Conclusion: Patients from the MOMENTUM-3 randomized trial were considered for this observational follow-up study, per-protocol analyses found that receipt of a fully magnetically levitated centrifugal-flow LVAD versus axial-flow LVAD was associated with a better composite outcome and higher likelihood of overall survival at 5 years. Findings of present study support the use of the fully magnetically levitated LVAD.

ARTICLE COMMENTARY

The estimated prevalence of heart failure in India is about 8–10 million individuals with an annual mortality of 1–1.6 lakh.[1] Patients with refractory heart failure have a poor quality of life and a grave prognosis with 1-year mortality up to 35–40%. Hence, advanced heart failure can be fatal without the use of inotropes, mechanical support devices like extracorporeal membrane oxygenation (ECMO) or Impella, heart transplantation or durable left ventricular assist devices (LVADs). The first-generation axial flow LVADs (viz., HeartMate-2) has proven 48% superiority over medical therapy as per the REMATCH trial.[2] But, experience from the USA and India on the HeartMate-2 axial flow devices has shown a stroke rate of about 19% and a 2-year survival rate of 76%. The New Generation HeartMate-3 Centrifugal Pump which uses a bearingless, low shear blood flow and magnetically levitation technology has shown a much improved 2-year survival of 83%, low pump thrombosis rates (1,2%) and much lower stroke rate of <10% and 78% event-free survival at 2 years. These observations have been elegantly demonstrated in the MOMENTUM-3 trial on 1,028 LVAD implanted patients (519 on HeartMate-3 and 513 on HeartMate-2 pumps) and of which 825 patients were in cardiogenic shock.[3] This study showed a significant clinical advantage of the HM3 LVAD over HM2 (77% of patients free of any events vs. 64.8%). The Follow-up study by Mehra et al. has shown a 5-year survival of 58.4% in the HeartMate-3 group with a much-reduced incidence of stroke, bleeding, or pump thrombosis.[3] This study surely goes a long way in establishing the life-saving role of durable implantable LV assist pumps for patients with advanced heart failure and cardiogenic shock and adds to the available tools for treating sick heart failure patients in India.

ARTICLE 2

Right Heart Failure Following Left Ventricular Device Implantation: Natural History, Risk Factors, and Outcomes: An Analysis of the STS INTERMACS Database

Kapelios CJ, Lund LH, Wever-Pinzon O, Selzman CH, Myers SL, Cantor RS, et al. Right Heart Failure Following Left Ventricular Device Implantation: Natural History, Risk Factors, and Outcomes: An Analysis of the STS INTERMACS Database.
Circ Heart Fail. 2022;15(6):e008706.

Abstract

Background: Limited studies to date were available for right heart failure (RHF) post-left ventricular assist device (LVAD). Currently, a new definition of RHF was introduced Interagency Registry for Mechanically Assisted Circulatory Support. On the basis of this definition, the present study is designed to investigate the natural history, risk factors, and outcomes of post-LVAD RHF.

Methods: From June 2, 2014 to June 30, 2016, patients registered in the Interagency Registry for Mechanically Assisted Circulatory Support/Society of Thoracic Surgeons Database and implanted with continuous flow LVAD were included in this study. Here, we assessed RHF incidence and predictors, survival after RHF. Elevated central venous pressure, peripheral edema, ascites, and use of inotropes are the manifestations of RHF which were separately analyzed.

Results: Prevalence of 1-month RHF was 24% among 5,537 LVAD recipients (mean 57 ± 13 years, 49% destination therapy, support 18.9 months). Out of these, in 5.3% RHF persisted at 12 months. On the other hand, de novo RHF occurred in 5.1% when first identified at 3 months and persisted at 12 months in 17% of patients and at 6 months occurred in 4.8% and persisted at 12 months in 25%. Risk factors for RHC incidence at 3 months represented by higher preimplant blood urea nitrogen (OR 1.03 –1.09 per 5 mg/dL increase; $p < 0.0001$), previous tricuspid valve repair/replacement (OR 2.01–10.09; $p < 0.001$), severely depressed right ventricular systolic function (OR 1.17–2.20; $p = 0.004$); and centrifugal versus axial LVAD (OR 1.15–1.78; $p = 0.001$). The lowest 2-year survival (57%) was noted in patients with persistent RHF at 3 months while patients with de novo RHF or RHF which resolved by 3 months had shown more favorable survival outcomes (75% and 78% at 2 years, respectively; $p < 0.001$).

Conclusion: A common and frequently transient condition, RHF at 1 or 3 months post-LVAD was, if resolved, associated with a relatively favorable prognosis. On the contrary, de novo, more frequently occurred persistent disorder was a late RHF post-LVAD (>6 months) and it was found to be associated with increased mortality. For RHF assessment and risk stratification in LVAD recipients the 1-, 3-, and 6-month time points may be used.

ARTICLE COMMENTARY

After durable left ventricular (LV) assist implantation, there remains a 10–40% risk of development of right heart failure. The genesis of right ventricular failure is multifactorial which includes increased systemic venous inflow into the right ventricle, leftward shift of interventricular septum (IVS) due to emptying of the left ventricle, cardiopulmonary bypass relates right ventricular (RV) dysfunction, increased pulmonary vascular resistance or worsening tricuspid regurgitation. Many studies also have developed preoperative risk scores for the development of postoperative RV failure like central venous pressure (CVP)/pulmonary capillary wedge pressure (PCWP) ratio of >0.63, need for preoperative ventilatory support, blood urea nitrogen (BUN) >39 mg/dL,[4] high right atrial (RA) pressure >15 mm, RV ejection fraction <30%, RA dimension >50 mm and severe tricuspid regurgitation.[5] The Michigan risk score considers four variables creatinine >2.4 mg/dL, bilirubin >2 mg/dL, SGOT >80 IU/dL, and vasopressor use.[6] The large STS-INTERMACS (the Society of Thoracic Surgeons-the Interagency Registry for Mechanically Assisted Circulatory Support) database of the large 5,537 LVAD recipients is an important advance in the knowledge regarding clinically important variables for the risk of RHF. The variables identified were preoperative tricuspid regurgitation, right ventricular dysfunction, left ventricular ejection fraction (LVEF) <20%, higher systemic blood pressure, higher body surface area, and slight higher incidence noted with centrifugal LVADs. These factors can be ameliorated by careful preoperative patient selection, preoperative use of inotropes like milrinone or levosimendan, control of blood pressure, and perioperative management of pulmonary vascular resistance. Right ventricular failure in the postoperative period is managed by early use of right ventricular assist devices like temporary surgical CENTRIMAG RVADs, Impella RP, or insertion of a bi-lumen PROTEK DUO cannula with external pump support. But, the STS study also shows that persistent RV failure beyond 6 months carries a worse prognosis. This area of right ventricular failure after LVADs is hence clinically important and such studies like STS INTERMACS database are an important advance in this area.

ARTICLE 3

Renal Sympathetic Denervation in Patients with Heart Failure with Preserved Ejection Fraction

Kresoja KP, Rommel KP, Fengler K, von Roeder M, Besler C, Lücke C, et al. Renal Sympathetic Denervation in Patients With Heart Failure With Preserved Ejection Fraction.
Circ Heart Fail. 2021;14(3):e007421.

Abstract

Background: The most common comorbidity in patients with heart failure with preserved ejection fraction (HFpEF) is arterial hypertension which mediates adverse hemodynamics through related aortic stiffness and increased pulsatile load. The present study is designed to examine the clinical and hemodynamic implications of renal sympathetic denervation (RDN) in HFpEF patients and uncontrolled arterial hypertension.

Methods: In a single-center patients undergoing RDN from 2011 to 2018 were retrospectively analyzed and classified as HFpEF ($n = 99$) or no HF ($n = 65$). Through cardiac magnetic resonance imaging stroke volume index and aortic distensibility were measured, and left ventricular (LV) systolic and echocardiographically assessed diastolic properties.

Results: Patients with HFpEF had shown higher stroke volume index [median 40 (interquartile range 33–48) vs. 33 (26–40) mL/m^2, $p = 0.002$], pulse pressure [69 (63–77) vs. 61 (55–67) mm Hg, $p < 0.001$], but lower LV-VPES$_{100 \text{ mm Hg}}$ [18 (10–28) vs. 24 (15–40) mL, $p = 0.007$] and aortic distensibility [1.5 (1.1–2.6) vs. 2.7 (1.1–3.5) 10^{-3} mm Hg^{-1}, $p = 0.013$] as compared to no-HF patients at baseline. On comparing patients with HFpEF and no-HF patients following RDN [−9 (−16 to −2), $p < 0.001$] decreased systolic blood pressure was noted. In HFpEF patients after RDN stroke volume index [−3 (−9 to +3) mL/m^2, $p = 0.011$] was observed to be decreased and aortic distensibility [0.2 (−0.1 to +1.1) 10^{-3} mm Hg^{-1}, $p = 0.007$) and systolic stiffness ($p < 0.001$) were increased. Also, observed decrease in LV diastolic stiffness and LV filling pressures as well as NT-proBNP (N-terminal pro-B-type natriuretic peptide) after RDN in patients with HFpEF ($p = 0.032$, $p = 0.043$, and $p < 0.001$, respectively).

Conclusion: Increased stroke volume index, vascular, and LV stiffness were shown by patients with HFpEF undergoing RDN in comparison to no-HF patients. RDN might be a potential therapeutic strategy for arterial hypertension and HFpEF as following RDN those hemodynamic alterations and reduced systolic and diastolic LV stiffness were partly normalized.

ARTICLE COMMENTARY

Present study was planned to inspect the clinical and hemodynamic effects of renal sympathetic denervation (RDN) in patients with arterial hypertension (aHT) and heart failure with preserved ejection fraction (HFpEF) as compared to patients without HF. This was a retrospective observational study, in which data was collected from group of patients >18 years who undertook RDN at a single high-volume center from a period of 2011–2018. All patients were post hoc graded as HFpEF or no HF by following the guidelines provided by the European Society of Cardiology. Individually, selective patients who were presented with uncontrolled aHT were considered for present analysis, no redo RDN procedures were involved. After RDN, medication prescribed had to be steady for >4 weeks before and was anticipated to remain unchanged. 115 out of the total enrolled patients underwent radiofrequency ablation (Medtronic, Minnesota, MN), and 49 patients subjected for ultrasound RDN (Paradise, ReCor Medical, Palo Alto, CA). BP reductions of ≥5 mm Hg in patients at daytime ambulatory blood pressure monitoring

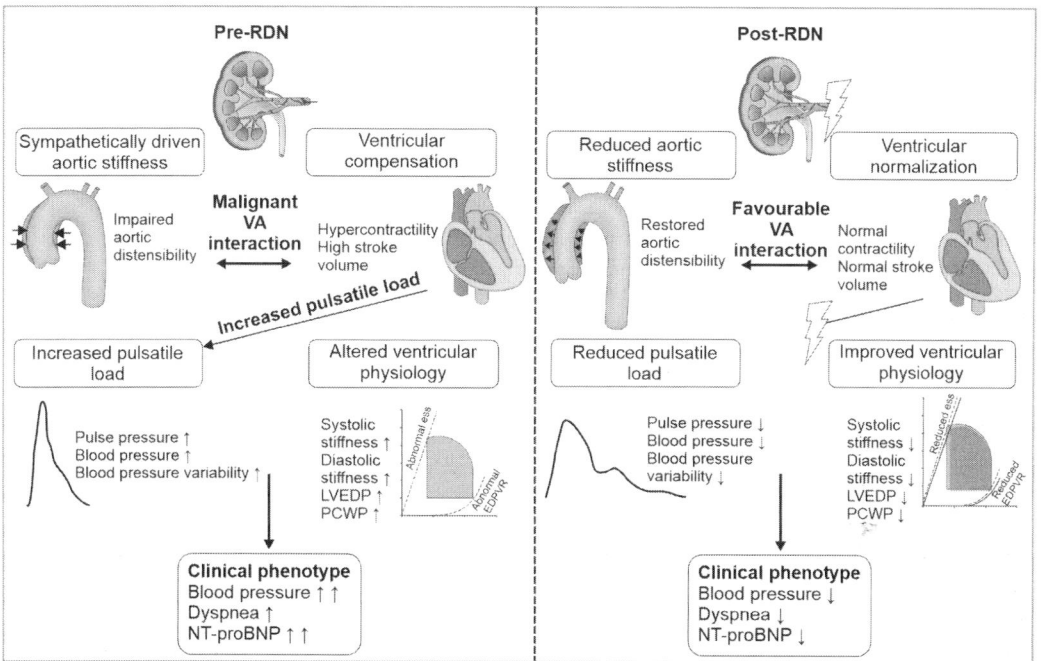

FIG. 1: Comparison between pre- and postrenal sympathetic denervation (RDN).

(LVEDP: left ventricular end-diastolic pressure; NT-proBNP: N-terminal pro-brain natriuretic peptide; PCWP: pulmonary capillary wedge pressure; RDN: renal sympathetic denervation)

(ABPM) after duration of 3 months were called as responders. The BP > 135 mm Hg on systolic and <85 mm Hg on diastolic were considered as isolated systolic hypertension on daytime ABPM.

Suggested beneficial mechanism of renal sympathetic denervation in patients with HFpEF **(Fig. 1)**.

In cohort of an uncontrolled aHT, patients showing HFpEF are categorized by factors like state of hypercontractility, increased aortic stiffness in addition to pathological ventriculo-arterial interaction. In patients with HFpEF, a similar BP reduction and no HF; also, a reversal of adverse hemodynamic alterations in HFpEF patients with improvements in LV filling characteristics and pressures was witnessed after RDN. Thus, RDN may become a promising treatment choice on getting a hypertensive HFpEF phenotype, which further permits for investigations in a prospective randomized controlled trial.

ARTICLE 4

Renal Compression in Heart Failure: The Renal Tamponade Hypothesis

Boorsma EM, Ter Maaten JM, Voors AA, van Veldhuisen DJ. Renal Compression in Heart Failure: The Renal Tamponade Hypothesis.
JACC Heart Fail. 2022;10(3):175-83.

Abstract

One of the strongest predictors of outcome in heart failure (HF) is renal dysfunction. Numerous studies have discovered that worse condition of renal function in HF is contributed by both reduced perfusion and increased congestion (and central venous pressure). The present article advises the presence of a novel factor relating to cardiac and renal dysfunction: "renal tamponade" or compression of renal structures caused by the limited space for expansion. The described space can be limited either by the rigid renal capsule that encloses the renal interstitial tissue or by the layer of fat around the kidneys or by exerting pressure by the peritoneal space on the retroperitoneal kidneys. Effective alleviating of pressure-related injury within the kidney itself is shown by renal decapsulation in many animal models of HF and acute renal ischemia, therefore, supporting this concept in HF making it a potentially interesting novel treatment strategy.

ARTICLE COMMENTARY

Present paper advises a novel factor in the correlation between cardiac and renal dysfunction: "renal tamponade" or compression of renal structures occurred due to availability of the limited space for expansion. This space can be limited either by the rigid renal capsule that encloses the renal interstitial tissue or by the layer of fat around the kidneys or by the peritoneal space exerting pressure on the retroperitoneal kidneys. In year 1990, it was revealed that the human kidney is very sensitive to changes in perfusion conditions so much, that decrease in cardiac index by 25% results in decrease in renal blood flow by as much as 50%. Many studied groups of numerous research presented that reduced renal perfusion is one of the strongest determinants of glomerular filtration rate (GFR) in heart failure (HF).

Additionally, tubules and glomeruli, veins are also affected by intracapsular pressure overload, as has been confirmed in numerous small ultrasound studies in humans. In animal models of HF and acute renal ischemia, renal decapsulation revealed to be effective in improving pressure-related injury within the kidney itself, as a result supporting this perception and makes it as a potentially remarkable novel treatment in HF. About >100 years old data was available on decapsulation in humans. Renal capsular incision or full decapsulation was a preferred treatment frequently performed for various indications, ranging from renal abscesses to preeclampsia and oliguria, but not congestive HF, in the late 19th and early 20th centuries. Healthier alternatives listed, such as dialysis and antibiotic treatment, in addition to challenging results on the benefit of decapsulation on renal outcomes, ultimately rendered renal decapsulation obsolete in situations of acute kidney injury. Here, the authors recommend the renal tamponade hypothesis to better explain the inconsistent impairment in renal function in situations of increased central venous pressures in patients with HF. More research is required to reveal the connection between HF, congestion, obesity, and impaired renal function. Although, decreased renal perfusion may be challenging to manage, and indeed, attempts to improve renal perfusion have shown not to be associated with improved outcomes, intrarenal congestion may probably become a treatment target now. Thus, renal decompression therapies in future may be a novel therapeutic area to search for reducing the incidence of worsening renal function and worsening HF.

ARTICLE 5

Riociguat in Pulmonary Hypertension and Heart Failure with Preserved Ejection Fraction: The HemoDYNAMIC Trial

Dachs TM, Duca F, Rettl R, Binder-Rodriguez C, Dalos D, Ligios LC, et al. Riociguat in pulmonary hypertension and heart failure with preserved ejection fraction: the haemoDYNAMIC trial.
Eur Heart J. 2022;43(36):3402-13.

Abstract

Aims: The clinical course of heart failure with preserved ejection fraction (HFpEF) is severely aggravated by the presence of pulmonary hypertension (PH). To date, not yet-established therapies for heart failure and pulmonary vasodilators proved beneficial. The present study inspected the efficacy of chronic treatment with the oral soluble guanylate cyclase stimulator riociguat in patients with PH-HFpEF.

Methods and results: This is a phase IIb, multicenter, randomized, double-blind, placebo-controlled, parallel-group, DYNAMIC trial evaluated riociguat in PH-HFpEF. Across Austria and Germany, patients were recruited at five different hospitals. Mean pulmonary artery pressure ≥ 25 mm Hg, pulmonary arterial wedge pressure > 15 mm Hg, and left ventricular ejection fraction ≥ 50% were the key eligibility criteria for study subjects. With riociguat or placebo (1:1) patients were randomized to oral treatment. Initially, patients started at 0.5 mg three times daily (TID) and were uptitrated to 1.5 mg TID. Change from baseline to week 26 in cardiac output (CO) at rest was the primary efficacy endpoint, measured by right heart catheterization. On the full analysis set primary efficacy analyses were completed. A total of 58 patients received riociguat and 56 patients' placebo. In the riociguat group after 26 weeks, CO increased by 0.37 ± 1.263 L/min, and in the placebo group decreased by −0.11 ± 0.921 L/min (least-squares mean difference: 0.54 L/min; 95% CI 0.112, 0.971; $p = 0.0142$). Dropped out five patients due to riociguat-related adverse events, but not reported riociguat-related serious adverse event or death happened.

Conclusion: The vasodilator riociguat proved to play an important role in the improvement of hemodynamics in PH-HFpEF. In most patients, riociguat was considered safe but headed more dropouts as compared to placebo, and no change in clinical symptoms was observed within the study period.

ARTICLE COMMENTARY

The clinical course of heart failure with preserved ejection fraction (HFpEF) is severely aggravated by pulmonary hypertension (PH). Till date, any of the neither traditional heart failure therapies nor pulmonary vasodilators evidenced favorable in these two entities presenting concomitantly.

The DYNAMIC study inspected the efficacy of chronic treatment with the oral soluble guanylate cyclase stimulator riociguat in patients with PH-HFpEF. The main eligibility criteria followed to include the patients were mean pulmonary artery pressure ≥25 mm Hg, pulmonary arterial wedge pressure >15 mm Hg, and left ventricular ejection fraction ≥50%. Patients were considered for randomization to give oral treatment with riociguat or placebo (1:1). Patients initially started at 0.5 mg three times daily (TID) and were uptitrated to 1.5 mg TID.

Riociguat proved to be shown improvement in CO at rest with a placebo-corrected change from a baseline of 0.54 L/min. Here we find significant positive hemodynamic effects of riociguat, also witnessed prove regarding decreased pulmonary vascular resistance (PVR) and transpulmonary pressure gradient (TPG), and stability of systemic vascular resistance (SVR) and pulmonary arterial wedge pressure (PAWP). The detected hemodynamic changes were not convoyed by significant improvements in N-terminal pro-brain natriuretic peptide (NT-proBNP) serum levels, WHO functional class (WHO-FC), exercise capacity, or quality of life (QOL). Generally, riociguat had a promising safety profile. In both treatment groups, greatest TEAEs (Treatment Emergent Adverse Events) were found to be mild or moderate intensity. The utmost frequent TEAEs were observed to be peripheral edema (riociguat: 29.3%; placebo: 30.4%), dyspnea (riociguat: 25.9%; placebo: 21.4%), and hypotension (riociguat: 22.4%; placebo: 12.5%). Nineteen (32.8%) study drug-related TEAEs ensued with riociguat and 12 (21.4%) with placebo. Hypertension was the majorly reported condition for drug-related study on TEAE for both treatments. Drug–drug interactions have been previously reported for riociguat and direct oral anticoagulants (DOACs) which are responsible for bioaccumulation and excessive bleeding conditions. As compared to the placebo group drop-out rates were higher for patients in the riociguat. This variance happened due to reasons like higher rates of initial intolerance, nontolerable adverse events (AEs), and withdrawal of consent but no changes in clinical symptoms were noted within the study period. Whether clinically meaningful endpoints of morbidity and mortality influenced by treatment vary with riociguat merits, for this further investigation in adequately designed trials are needed for clarifications. The current patient population of this study was elderly representative; predominantly female HFpEF population with invasively confirmed PH. DYNAMIC is the first study to evaluate the hemodynamic and clinical effects of chronic treatment with the use of oral soluble guanylate cyclase (sGC) stimulator riociguat. Overall, with respect to patients who completed the study riociguat had shown a favorable safety profile. Yet, higher dropout rates claim careful monitoring in future trials. Undoubtedly, patients enrolled in DYNAMIC demonstrated a different subtype of PH with less severe hemodynamic changes as compared to precapillary PH collectives. Moreover, there are some limitations of DYNAMIC trial as it was not powered to detect any clinical changes in patients and these factors need to be considered regarding the interpretation of results. In respect of the previous reported neutral trials of other sGC stimulators in HFpEF, it is difficult to tell how the results of DYNAMIC, showing a hemodynamic effect, will change the landscape of treatment. In conclusion, riociguat observed to show improvement in cardiac output (CO), pulmonary vascular resistance (PVR), and further pulmonary hemodynamics, and was safe in most patients with PH-HFpEF, but there are more dropouts and did not change any clinical symptoms within the study period. Whether clinically meaningful endpoints of morbidity and mortality may be influenced by treatment with riociguat merits, so further investigation in adequately designed trials are needed.

ARTICLE 6

Randomized Trial of Targeted Transendocardial Mesenchymal Precursor Cell Therapy in Patients with Heart Failure

Perin EC, Borow KM, Henry TD, Mendelsohn FO, Miller LW, Swiggum E, et al. Randomized Trial of Targeted Transendocardial Mesenchymal Precursor Cell Therapy in Patients With Heart Failure.
J Am Coll Cardiol. 2023;81(9):849-63.

Abstract

Background: In patients of heart failure with reduced ejection fraction (HFrEF) have shown improved outcomes by allogeneic mesenchymal precursor cells (MPCs), these are immunoselected cells with anti-inflammatory properties.

Objectives: Present study was planned to evaluate the efficacy and safety of MPCs in patients with high-risk HFrEF.

Methods: This is a randomized, double-blind, multicenter study considered a single transendocardial administration procedure of MPCs or sham-control in 565 intention-to-treat patients with HFrEF on guideline-directed therapies. Outcomes like time-to-recurrent events caused by decompensated HFrEF or successfully resuscitated symptomatic ventricular arrhythmias are the primary endpoint of the study. The components of the primary endpoint were included in hierarchical secondary endpoints, which are time-to-first terminal cardiac events, and all-cause death. For myocardial infarction or stroke or cardiovascular death, a distinct and composite major adverse cardiovascular events analysis was performed. Echocardiography was done at baseline and at 12 months. For disease severity, baseline plasma high-sensitivity C-reactive protein levels were estimated.

Results: Similar primary endpoint and secondary endpoints, as were terminal cardiac events noted between treatment groups (HR 1.17; 95% CI 0.81–1.69; $p = 0.41$). In patients with inflammation in comparison with control subjects, MPCs increased left ventricular ejection fraction from baseline to 12 months was observed. Observed a decrease in the risk of myocardial infarction or stroke by 58% (HR 0.42; 95% CI 0.23–0.76) by MPCs and the risk of three-point major adverse cardiovascular events by 28% (HR 0.72; 95% CI 0.51–1.03) in the analysis population ($n = 537$), and by 75% (HR 0.25; 95% CI 0.09–0.66) and 38% (HR 0.62; 95% CI 0.39–1.00), respectively, in patients with inflammation (baseline high-sensitivity C-reactive protein ≥2 mg/L).

Conclusion: Results of the trial showed the observation for the primary and secondary endpoints of the study were negative. MPCs may improve outcomes suggested by positive signals in prespecified, and post hoc exploratory analyses, particularly in patients with inflammation.

ARTICLE COMMENTARY

Patients with heart failure with reduced ejection fraction (HFrEF) have still high morbidity and mortality despite advances in pharmacotherapy. The two most important determinants in the pathophysiologic progression of HF are neurohormonal activation and underlying inflammation. The present-day guideline-directed medical therapy (GDMT) targets neurohormonal activation but acute and chronic inflammation which initiates multiple pathophysiological pathways, factors, and processes remains to be addressed or has not shown clinically significant benefit.

Mesenchymal precursor cells (MPCs) are allogeneic, immunoselected cells with anti-inflammatory properties that are obtained from human bone marrow mononuclear cell populations. Using proprietary techniques, these immunoselected cells were culture extended and can be stored in liquid nitrogen until use. MPCs have been shown in preclinical studies to decrease macrophage-dependent inflammation and advances microvascular blood flow through the release of multiple critical angiogenic factors that act in concert to make microvascular capillary networks in ischemic tissues. These factors also reduce proinflammatory cytokines responsible for an increased endothelial nitric oxide synthase activity, nitric oxide bioavailability, and reversed the endothelial dysfunction. Hence, MPCs proved to have the potential to improve myocardial perfusion and contractility despite the fact of reversing cardiac and systemic endothelial dysfunction. Therefore, this study was designed to assess the efficacy and safety of MPCs in high-risk HFrEF patients. It was randomized, double-blind, multicenteric study which assessed a single transendocardial administration procedure of MPCs or sham-control in 565 intention-to-treat patients with HFrEF on prescribed guideline-directed therapies. The location for cell delivery was identified by left ventricular (LV) electrical mapping of viable but electrically abnormal myocardium using the NOGA Cardiac Navigational System in combination with the NogaStar Mapping Catheter (Johnson and Johnson). To deliver approximately 150 million MPCs in 15–20 injection sites (in 0.2 mL volume containing 8–10 million MPCs) the MyoStar injection catheter was preferred. Till date this was one of the biggest clinical trials of cell therapy in HFrEF. The primary endpoint of the study was time-to-recurrent events caused by decompensated HFrEF or successfully resuscitated symptomatic ventricular arrhythmias.

The secondary endpoints for the present study are basically components of the primary endpoint, time-to-first terminal cardiac events, and all-cause death. For this baseline and 12-month echocardiography was done. Baseline plasma high-sensitivity C-reactive protein (hsCRP) levels were estimated to know disease severity. The primary endpoints of the study are reduction in recurrent nonfatal hospitalization of these patients or urgent care events due to decompensated heart failure or successfully resuscitated high-grade symptomatic ventricular arrhythmias. The associated main secondary endpoints were found to be negative. But, the MPCs increased LVEF from baseline to 12 months and also resulted in significant reductions in time to first event for myocardial infarction (MI) or stroke over an average follow-up time of 30 months, with the most improvement observed in patients with evidence of systemic inflammation (baseline hsCRP ≥ 2 mg/L). The improvement in LVEF appears to be driven predominantly by reductions in LV end-systolic volume. Improvement in early LV systolic function appears to strongly support MPCs' proposed mechanisms of action, which include improvement in the cardiac microvasculature with subsequent translation to LV systolic functional recovery and long-term reduction in major adverse cardiac events (MACE). The mechanisms of action of MPC therapy seems to be directed predominantly toward altering the inflammatory environment within the heart and the vasculature once the cells are activated by local tissue cytokines. In conclusion, in patients presented with heart failure and systemic inflammation transendocardial delivery of MPCs reduces MACE but does not avert hospitalization for decompensated heart failure or conditions of high-grade symptomatic ventricular arrhythmias.

ARTICLE 7

Cardiac Contractility Modulation Therapy Improves Health Status in Patients with Heart Failure with Preserved Ejection Fraction: A Pilot Study (CCM-HFpEF)

Linde C, Grabowski M, Ponikowski P, Rao I, Stagg A, Tschöpe C. Cardiac contractility modulation therapy improves health status in patients with heart failure with preserved ejection fraction: a pilot study (CCM-HFpEF). *Eur J Heart Fail.* 2022;24(12):2275-84.

Abstract

Aims: Present study is intended to estimate the potential benefits of cardiac contractility modulation (CCM) in patients with heart failure with preserved ejection fraction (HFpEF).

Methods and results: The present study was a prospective, multicenter, single-arm, pilot study of CCM therapy in patients with HFpEF and New York Heart Association (NYHA) class II or III. In an Echo Core Laboratory, echocardiographic parameters were measured to decide study eligibility. Patients were followed for 24 weeks after CCM device implantation. A total of 47 patients (mean age 74.3 ± 4.4 years, 70.2% female) were enrolled, with left ventricular ejection fraction of 59 ± 4.4%, 63.8% with hypertension, 46.8% with atrial fibrillation, 40.4% with diabetes, 31.9% with at least one heart failure hospitalization in the prior year, 61.7% in NYHA class III, and 48.9 ± 21.7 summary score of Kansas City Cardiomyopathy Questionnaire (KCCQ). There was an event-free rate of 93.6% for the primary safety endpoint (device- and procedure-related complications), as adjudicated by an independent physician committee also, the primary efficacy endpoint (mean change in the KCCQ overall summary score) was improved by 18.0 ± 16.6 points ($p < 0.001$).

Conclusion: The benefits of CCM may be advantageous to the HFpEF patient population demonstrated by the present study. Observing the significant improvement in health status, without any impact on safety, supports that utilization of CCM for patients with HFpEF could prove to be encouraging.

ARTICLE COMMENTARY

The treatment of heart failure with reduced ejection fraction (HFrEF) has seen many novel therapies in the last decade which were well-proven in clinical trials whereas treatment for heart failure with preserved ejection fraction (HFpEF) is evolving. Cardiac contractility modulation (CCM) therapy has been shown to be a promising alternative in patients of HFrEF who remain symptomatic in spite of guideline-directed medical therapy (GDMT). CCM is a device-based therapy that includes application of relatively high-voltage (≈ 7.5 V), long-duration (≈ 20 milliseconds), biphasic electric signals to the right ventricular septal wall during the absolute myocardial refractory period. These signals influence the biology of the failing myocardium and induce an acute and mild augmentation of left ventricular (LV) contractile strength without an increase in myocardial oxygen consumption.

Initial studies of CCM in HFrEF patients have shown improvement in peak oxygen uptake (VO_2), New York Heart Association (NYHA) class, health status, and 6-minute walk distance (6MWD) difference in patients with higher baseline left ventricular ejection fraction (LVEF) and therefore this pilot study was conducted in patients with HFpEF. The included patients were in NYHA class II or III despite receiving optimal medical therapy and N-terminal pro-brain natriuretic peptide (NT-proBNP) >220 pg/mL for subjects in sinus rhythm or >600 pg/mL for subjects in atrial fibrillation. Echocardiography inclusion criteria were left atrial volume index (LAVi) ≥34 mL/m² or LVH >12 mm and either E/e′ ≥13 or septal e′ <7 cm/s or lateral e′ <10 cm/s. Overall 47 patients from Europe and Australia were enrolled and after CCM implantation was followed for 24 weeks. The primary efficacy endpoint of the study was a mean change in health status as measured by the Kansas City Cardiomyopathy Questionnaire (KCCQ), overall summary score from baseline to 24 weeks following the CCM device implant were recorded. The secondary efficacy endpoints are to record the mean change from baseline to 24 weeks of NYHA class, NT-proBNP, and echocardiographic parameters like LAVi, septal E' velocity, and septal E/E' ratio.

The result revealed a significant improvement in the KCCQ score of 18.0 ± 16.6 points ($p < 0.001$) with or without atrial fibrillation. NYHA class improved by 0.5 ± 0.6 whereas the median NT-proBNP at 24 weeks increased by 23.0 pg/mL from baseline ($p = 0.077$), which symbolizes a marginally significant increase. Echocardiography parameters shown marginal improvements in the mean LAVi (–2.8 ± 8.2 mL/m^2, $p = 0.034$) and septal E/e' (–0.9 ± 4.7, $p = 0.038$) while septal e' remained unchanged. The primary safety endpoint analysis showed an event-free rate of 93.6% with no serious adverse events (SAEs) reported deemed as having a possible, probable, or causal relationship with the CCM device. In conclusion, this pilot study has shown that CCM therapy may show significant improvement in health position for patients with HFpEF while providing the same safety profile as formerly seen in those patients who were receiving CCM therapy with systolic dysfunction. There are major limitations of the study which include the factors such as small sample size, single-arm design without control group inclusion. Therefore, a larger study is needed before giving any firm recommendation for CCM therapy in clinical practice.

ARTICLE 8

Baroreflex Activation Therapy with the Barostim™ Device in Patients with Heart Failure with Reduced Ejection Fraction: A Patient Level Meta-analysis of Randomized Controlled Trials

Coats AJS, Abraham WT, Zile MR, Lindenfeld JA, Weaver FA, Fudim M, et al. Baroreflex activation therapy with the Barostim™ device in patients with heart failure with reduced ejection fraction: a patient level meta-analysis of randomized controlled trials.
Eur J Heart Fail. 2022;24(9):1665-73.

Abstract

Aims: The association of heart failure with reduced ejection fraction (HFrEF) with high morbidity and mortality, poor quality of life (QOL), and significant exercise limitation was already acknowledged. Adverse prognosis and symptoms in HFrEF predicted by sympathovagal imbalance, so far it has not been specifically targeted by any guideline-recommended device therapy to date. The first neuromodulation technology approved by Food and Drug Administration for HFrEF is Barostim™, which directly addresses the above-described imbalance. The present study aimed to examine all randomized trial evidence to assess the effect of baroreflex activation therapy (BAT) on heart failure symptoms, QOL, and N-terminal pro-brain natriuretic peptide (NT-proBNP) in HFrEF.

Methods and results: On all appropriate trials that randomized HFrEF patients to BAT + guideline-directed medical therapy (GDMT) or GDMT alone (open-label) for individual patient data (IPD) meta-analysis was performed. Parameters that contain 6-month changes in 6-minute hall walk (6MHW) distance, Minnesota Living With Heart Failure (MLWHF) QOL score, NT-proBNP, and New York Heart Association (NYHA) class in all patients and three subgroups were the included endpoints. This study included a total of 554 randomized patients. BAT provided significant improvement in 6MHW distance of 49 m [95% confidence interval (CI) 33, 64], MLWHF QOL of –13 points (95% CI –17, –10), and 3.4 higher odds of improving at least one NYHA class (95% CI 2.3, 4.9) when comparing from baseline to 6 months in all patients. Observed similar improvements in the above-described parameter, or found better, in patients who showed baseline NT-proBNP <1,600 pg/mL, regardless of the cardiac resynchronization therapy indication status.

Conclusion: Baroreflex activation therapy improves exercise capacity NYHA class, and QOL in HFrEF patients receiving GDMT suggested by an IPD meta-analysis. Across the range of studies, patients with the above-described clinical parameters were found to be meaningful improvements. In subjects with a lower baseline, NT-proBNP BAT was observed to be associated with an improvement in NT-proBNP.

ARTICLE COMMENTARY

In the last decade, there has been a major breakthrough in the pharmacological management of patients with heart failure with reduced ejection fraction (HFrEF). But, in spite of all these developments, many patients remain symptomatic in NYHA functional class II–III. The role of autonomic imbalance with increased activity of the sympathetic nervous system along with under activity of the parasympathetic nervous system has been studied in patients with HFrEF in the last few years. This autonomic imbalance exacerbates renal salt and water retention, peripheral vasoconstriction, and cardiac remodeling which contributes to symptom persistence and progression, disease progression, and increases the risk of mortality and HF hospitalizations. The present approved pharmacotherapy in HF like β-blockers, mineralocorticoid receptor antagonists, and renin–angiotensin–aldosterone system inhibitors modulate the autonomic system but indirectly and also have no effect on the parasympathetic or reflex system.

Baroreflex activation therapy (BAT) with CVRx® BarostimNEO™ system is the first neuromodulation device that directly modulates the cardiac autonomic system in patients of HFrEF in NYHA class II and III. It has been studied in two multicenter randomized trials (Phase II HOPE4HF and Phase III BeAT-HF). The device activates the baroreflex and produces autonomic modulation by inhibiting cardiac sympathetic outflow and activating the parasympathetic nervous system. The BarostimNEO™ system has two components: A carotid sinus lead surgically placed on the outside of the carotid sinus and an implantable pulse generator (IPG) placed in the subcutaneous pocket below the clavicle-like pacemaker. The lead is tunneled over the clavicle to the IPG.

The meta-analysis of the two trials included a total number of 554 patients with HFrEF (LVEF < 35%), NYHA class II or III and on guideline-directed medical therapy (GDMT) and was randomized 1:1 to either GDMT (Control) or BAT + GDMT (BAT). The endpoints were changed in Minnesota Living With Heart Failure (MLWHF) QOL score, NYHA class, 6-minute hall walk distance (6MHW), and N-terminal pro-brain natriuretic peptide (NT-proBNP) at 6 months. The meta-analysis revealed treatment with BAT was safe and demonstrated significant improvement in MLWHF QOL of –13 points, 3.4 higher odds of improving at least one NYHA class, 6MHW distance of 49 m, and NT-proBNP/BNP at the end of 6-month. The improvements in endpoints at 6-month were significant in patients with baseline NT-proBNP < 1,600 pg/mL regardless of the cardiac resynchronization therapy indication status. This differential benefit in patients with NT-proBNP < 1,600 pg/mL may be due to advanced disease in patients with NT-proBNP > 1,600 pg/mL. The higher level of natriuretic peptides correlates with greater left ventricular mass, worse left ventricular diastolic dysfunction, and higher pulmonary pressure, as well as a higher prevalence of comorbidities such as renal dysfunction and atrial fibrillation. BAT has shown benefit in all subgroups of patients with the most pronounced benefit in patients with NT-proBNP < 1,600 pg/mL and no indications for CRT. The therapeutic effects of BAT were more impressive in females whereas traditional pharmacotherapy has less benefit as compared to males. This may be because, in women of advanced age, the sympathetic baroreflex sensitivity decreases more so than in men of similar age.

The main challenge with direct cardiac neuromodulation in comparison to pharmacotherapy is the lack of clarity of optimal dosing like pulse amplitude and frequency and the nature of intervention delivery like intermittent or continuous delivery. The major limitation of this meta-analysis is the limited number of participants and open-label design. The long-term benefit of BAT will shed more light on the use of this first neuromodulation therapy in clinical practice.

REFERENCES

1. Chaturvedi V, Parakh N, Seth S, Bhargava B, Ramakrishnan S, Roy A, et al. Heart Failure in India: The INDUS study. J Pract Cardiovasc sci. 2016;2:28-35.
2. Rose EA, Gelijns AC, Moskowitz AJ, Heitjan DF, Stevenson LW, Dembitsky W, et al. Long Term use of a Left Ventricular Assist device for end stage Heart failure. N Engl J Med. 2001;345:1435-43.
3. Mehra MR, Uriel N, Naka Y, Cleveland JC Jr, Yuzefpolskaya M, Salerno CT, et al. A fully magnetically Levitated Left ventricular Assist device-Final report. N Engl J Med. 2019;380:1618-27.
4. Kormos RL, Teuteberg JJ, Pagani FD, Russell SD, John R, Miller LW, et al. Right ventricular failure in patient with the Heartmate II continuous-flow left ventricular assist device : incidence, risk factors, and effect on outcomes. J thorac Cardiovasc Surg. 2010;139:1316-24.
5. Potapov EV, Stepanenko A, Dandel M, Kukucka M, Lehmkuhl HB, Weng Y, et al. Tricuspid incompetence and geometry of right ventricle as predictors of right ventricle function after implantation of a left ventricular assist device. J Heart Lung Transplant. 2008;27:1275-81.
6. Matthews JC, Koelling TM, Pagani FD, Aaronson KD. The Right Ventricular failure risk score a preoperative tool for assessing the risk of RV failure in LV assist device candidates. J am Coll cardiol. 2008;51:2163-72.

SECTION 10

Interventions in Heart Failure

Section Editor: **PK Goel**

Co-Editors: Manik Chopra, Atul Kaushik

ARTICLE 1

Hospitalizations and Mortality in Patients with Secondary Mitral Regurgitation and Heart Failure: The COAPT Trial

Giustino G, Camaj A, Kapadia SR, Kar S, Abraham WT, Lindenfeld J, et al. Hospitalizations and Mortality in Patients With Secondary Mitral Regurgitation and Heart Failure: The COAPT Trial.
J Am Coll Cardiol. 2022;80(20):1857-68.

Abstract

Background: In patients presented with heart failure (HF) and severe secondary mitral regurgitation the impression of transcatheter edge-to-edge repair (TEER) on the rate and prognostic impression of hospitalizations is not clearly studied till date.

Objectives: This study was internationalized to assess the effect of the MitraClip™ percutaneous edge-to-edge repair system on fatal and nonfatal hospitalizations and also to discover their connection with mortality in the COAPT (Cardiovascular Outcomes Assessment of the MitraClip Percutaneous Therapy for Heart Failure Patients presented With Functional Mitral Regurgitation) trial.

Methods: Patients presented with HF (n = 614) with severe secondary mitral regurgitation were randomized according to TEER plus guideline-directed medical therapy (GDMT) versus GDMT alone. Hospitalizations were categorized as fatal if death happened during duration of hospitalization or considered nonfatal if the patient discharged status was stable and alive.

Results: TEER treatment, compared with GDMT alone, resulted in lower time-to-first-event rates of any heart failure hospitalization (HFH) (34.8% vs. 56.4%; HR 0.51; 95% CI 0.39–0.66) and fatal HFH (6.5% vs. 12.6%; HR 0.47; 95% CI 0.26–0.85) at 2 years. TEER also resulted in lesser incidence and rates of all-cause nonfatal and fatal hospitalizations. During the 2-year follow-up period, patients who underwent TEER expended an average of 2 more months alive and out of the hospital period than did patients who treated with GDMT alone (581 ± 27 days vs. 519 ± 26 days; $p = 0.002$). All HFHs (adjusted HR 6.37; 95% CI 4.63–8.78) and nonfatal HFHs (adjusted HR 1.78; 95% CI 1.27–2.49) were consistently independently associated with increased 2-year mortality in both the TEER and GDMT groups ($p_{interaction}$ = 0.34 and 0.39, respectively).

Conclusion: Compared with GDMT alone, patients presented with HF and severe secondary mitral regurgitation undergoing TEER with the percutaneous edge-to-edge repair system had poorer 2-year rates of fatal and nonfatal all-cause hospitalizations rates and HFH and observed that they spent more time being alive and out of the hospital course, in the COAPT trial. Regardless of treatment HFHs were strongly associated with mortality.

ARTICLE COMMENTARY

Patients with heart failure with reduced ejection fraction have a high mortality and poor clinical outcomes in the long term and this could be worse in the presence of significant mitral regurgitation (MR). Whether the reduction of MR through the transcatheter edge-to-edge repair (TEER) could reduce the adverse events in long-term follow is not well known. This study assessed the outcomes in patients with heart failure with reduced ejection fraction with significant secondary MR after TEER using the Abbott MitraClip.

The study was an open open-label multicenter randomized trial. The number of patients studied was 614 and the primary endpoints were all heart failure hospitalizations (fatal/nonfatal) and mortality with a follow-up period of 2 years postrandomization.

Ischemic/nonischemic cardiomyopathy with left ventricular ejection fraction (LVEF) between 20 and 50% and at least moderate to severe MR (3+/4+) in the New York Heart Association (NYHA) class II–Iva (ambulatory patients only) despite maximally tolerated GDMT and CRT if eligible were included. Really bad cases like ventricles with LVED (d) >7 cm were excluded so as to exclude the worst patients who would otherwise have very high mortality.

About 70% of all patients studied (TEER + GDMT/GDMT alone groups) were hospitalized during the course of the study for some reason or other showing the poor outcomes in these patients as a whole.

All-cause hospitalization (including fatal/nonfatal), however, was significantly less in the TEER group (68.6% vs. 80.7%, HR 0.76) ($p < 0.004$).

Nonheart failure-related hospitalizations, however, were no different in the two groups. HF hospitalization subgroup was more prone to subsequent mortality irrespective of the treatment group and mortality was higher with each successive hospitalization, as expected in a setting of worsening heart failure.

Transcatheter edge-to-edge repair resulted in 2 months longer time alive in the 2 years follow-up period.

In addition to treatment with TEER, several clinical variables suggestive of a more severe heart failure setting such as worse ECHO parameters, increased pulmonary artery (PA) pressure, increased left atrial (LA) size, increased B-type natriuretic peptide (BNP) values, low Kansas City Cardiomyopathy Questionnaire (KCCQ) scores, greater degrees of MR, and presence of atrial fibrillation (AF) were associated with increased HF hospitalizations and mortality. My inference of the trial is:

- TEER + GDMT might be better than GDMT alone, but the absolute long-term benefit is possibly small as on the whole, this is a group with poor long-term outcomes.
- This trial includes 614 patients from 78 centers which amounts to only 8 cases per center on average which means the majority of centers would be including

cases only in single digits. Hence, the operator's experience/expertise and the TEER result obtained in an individual case could be also a point to ponder upon rather than clubbing all cases together.

> **Key messages**
> - TEER is effective in reducing HF hospitalization and improving symptoms in patients with secondary MR and giving on extra lease of 2 months' longevity.
> - Patients with lesser severity of HF at baseline would have better outcomes independent of treatment strategy.
> - All heart failure hospitalized patients would have a higher mortality independent of study group.
> - Repeated HF hospitalization would be associated with worse fatal outcomes.

ARTICLE 2

Percutaneous Revascularization for Ischemic Left Ventricular Dysfunction

Perera D, Clayton T, O'Kane PD, Greenwood JP, Weerackody R, Ryan M, et al. Percutaneous Revascularization for Ischemic Left Ventricular Dysfunction.
Eur J Heart Fail. 2023;25(3):399-410.

Abstract

Background: Compared with optimal medical therapy (i.e., individually adjusted pharmacologic and device therapy for heart failure), whether revascularization by percutaneous coronary intervention (PCI) can improve event-free survival and left ventricular function in severe ischemic left ventricular systolic dysfunction patients, is not well understood.

Methods: In present study, patients with a left ventricular ejection fraction of 35% or less, extensive coronary artery disease responsive to PCI, and demonstrable myocardial viability to a strategy of either PCI plus optimal medical therapy (PCI group) or optimal medical therapy alone (optimal-medical-therapy group), are randomly assigned. The primary endpoint outcome was hospitalization for heart failure or death from any cause. Major secondary endpoints were left ventricular ejection fraction at 6 and 12 months and obtain scores for quality-of-life.

Results: Out of 700 patients who underwent randomization 347 were assigned to the PCI group and 353 to the optimal-medical-therapy group. A primary-outcome event happened in 129 patients (37.2%) in the PCI group and in 134 patients (38.0%) in the optimal-medical-therapy group [hazard ratio (HR) 0.99; 95% confidence interval (CI) 0.78–1.27; $p = 0.96$], over a time of 41 months. In the two groups at 6 months (mean difference −1.6 percentage points;

95% CI −3.7 to 0.5) and at 12 months (mean difference 0.9 percentage points; 95% CI −1.7 to 3.4) the left ventricular ejection fraction was similar. At 6 and 12 months, quality-of-life (QOL) scores appeared to favor the PCI group, but the difference had reduced at 24 months.

Conclusion: Revascularization by PCI did not result in a lower incidence of death from any cause or hospitalization for heart failure, among patients with severe ischemic left ventricular systolic dysfunction who received optimal medical therapy.

ARTICLE COMMENTARY

Ischemic left ventricular (LV) dysfunction is usually due to hibernating ischemic myocardium which could improve on revascularization, a concept that sounds logical and also has been shown to be true to some extent in patients undergoing coronary artery bypass grafting (CABG) as per the STICH trial on long-term (10 years) follow-up. Whether the same results could be replicated with percutaneous coronary intervention (PCI) is not known. The hypothesis of this study was to assess the PCI in patients with ischemic LV dysfunction with proven myocardial viability could have better event-free survival and show improved LV function at follow-up. Patients with LVEF < 35% with coronary artery disease (CAD) amicable to PCI and proven myocardial viability in the segments to be revascularized were randomized into PCI + GDMT versus GDMT alone. The primary endpoint included death from any cause and/or hospitalization for heart failure over a period of 2 years. The secondary endpoint was an improvement in left ventricular ejection fraction (LVEF) at 6/12 months. The total number of patients included was 700.

There was no difference in event-free survival in the two groups although quality-of-life (QOL) scores were better in the PCI group. The study concluded as a negative trial on the virtue of PCI having any benefit in patients with LV dysfunction.

■ VIEWPOINTS (MY THOUGHTS ON THE TRIAL)

It is not certain if there was a true association between coronary vessels revascularized and the viable segment location. Requirement as per the study of the protocol was based on the presence of only four viable segments which could very well be in territories not needing revascularization or not amicable to revascularization or failed revascularization (CTO, etc.). The percentage of cases with successful revascularization is not mentioned. Merely grouping into revascularization groups without successful intervention documented in the required vessel may not be beneficial. The majority of patients do not have angina in the study and we know PCI is largely a procedure to relieve angina. Recruitment of 700 cases over 40 centers over a period of 7 years (2013–2020) amounts to two cases/year/center which is nowhere close to real-world PCI practice. The involved case selection bias could be a factor responsible for the trial being negative. Also, changes in PCI technique over the years could play a role in this 10-year-long-drawn recruitment period study.

ARTICLE 3

Intermittent Occlusion of the Superior Vena Cava to Improve Hemodynamics in Patients with Acutely Decompensated Heart Failure: The VENUS-HF Early Feasibility Study

Kapur NK, Kiernan MS, Gorgoshvili I, Yousefzai R, Vorovich EE, Tedford RJ, et al. Intermittent Occlusion of the Superior Vena Cava to Improve Hemodynamics in Patients With Acutely Decompensated Heart Failure: The VENUS-HF Early Feasibility Study.
Circ Heart Fail. 2022;15(2):e008934.

Abstract

Background: A primary target of therapy for acutely decompensated heart failure remains reducing congestion. The first clinical trial testing for intermittent occlusion of the superior vena cava with the preCARDIA system is the VENUS-HF EFS (VENUS-Heart Failure Early Feasibility Study) to improve decongestion in acutely decompensated heart failure, a catheter mounted balloon and pump console were used.

Methods: This is a multicenter, prospective, single-arm exploratory safety and feasibility trial, for 12 or 24 hours 30 patients with acutely decompensated heart failure were assigned to preCARDIA therapy. Over 30 days obtain primary safety outcomes contain a combination of major adverse cardiovascular and cerebrovascular events. Secondary endpoints involved technical success well-defined as successful preCARDIA placement, treatment, and removal and reduction in right atrial and pulmonary capillary wedge pressure. Urine output and patient-reported symptoms are the other efficacy measures.

Results: A total of 30 patients were enrolled and assigned to receive the preCARDIA system. In 100% ($n = 30/30$) patients' freedom from device- or procedure-related major adverse events was observed. In 97% ($n = 29/30$) of patients, the system was successfully placed, activated, and removed after 12 ($n = 6$) or 24 hours ($n = 23$). The right atrial pressure was decreased by 34% (17 ± 4 vs. 11 ± 5 mm Hg, $p < 0.001$) and pulmonary capillary wedge pressure decreased by 27% (31 ± 8 vs. 22 ± 9 mm Hg, $p < 0.001$) when compared with baseline values. Urine output and net fluid balance increased by 130% and 156%, respectively, with up to 24 hours of treatment ($p < 0.01$), when compared with pretreatment values.

Conclusion: To reduce congestion in acutely decompensated heart failure, this is the new report for the first-in-human experience of intermittent superior vena cava occlusion using the preCARDIA system. Up to 24 hours PreCARDIA treatment was well tolerated without device- or procedure-related serious or major adverse events and associated with reduced filling pressures and increased urine output. These results of the present study support planning for future studies defining the clinical utility of the preCARDIA system.

ARTICLE COMMENTARY

Treating venous congestion, the hallmark of acute decompensated heart failure (ADHF), is the foremost strategy to decrease morbidity and mortality. Although diuretics are recommended, eventually after escalating doses, they develop resistance and cause neurohormonal activation and renal dysfunction. One novel approach is to reduce cardiac filling pressures by superior vena cava (SVC) through a catheter-mounted balloon occlusion and pump system, known as the preCARDIA system.

Kapur et al., in a prospective, multicenter, single-arm trial, the VENUS-HF study, tested the feasibility and safety of the precardiac system in patients with ADHF. The study mainly included patients 18–85 years of age presenting with ADHF, New York Heart Association class III–IV symptoms, and two or more signs of venous congestion with inadequate diuresis. The primary endpoint was freedom from the device or procedure-related major adverse events defined as death, myocardial infarction, major thromboembolic events, vascular damage requiring surgical intervention, hemorrhagic stroke, and prolongation of heart failure-related hospitalization. There were two secondary endpoints. First was acute technical success defined as successful device deployment, ability to deliver treatment, and successful removal of the device. Second, was a reduction in right atrial pressure (RAP) and pulmonary capillary wedge pressure (PCWP). The baseline hemodynamics and SVC patency assessment were done before the preCARDIA catheter was deployed in the pulmonary artery with a proximal balloon in SVC. SVC occlusion was done by inflating the balloon with dilated contrast which was confirmed by venogram and gradient assessment between RAP and internal jugular venous pressure. Intermittent occlusion was then done with a duty cycle of 5 minutes of occlusion followed by 30 seconds of deflation. The first six patients were treated for about 12 hours and after confirming safety, the remaining patients underwent about 24 hours occlusion therapy.

Among the 41 patients enrolled, 11 patients were excluded by screening and inadequate venous access. The device was successfully placed in 30 patients, but one patient could not be properly positioned so was excluded (acute technical success ~96.7%). The mean left ventricular ejection fraction was 27.5%, the mean RAP was 17.4 mm Hg, and the mean PCWP was 30.7 mm Hg. The primary end point was achieved in 100% of patients. Two deaths and two readmissions occurred in 30-day follow-up. Patients reported improvement in symptoms with no neurological deterioration or serious adverse events. RAP decreased by 34% and PCWP decreased by 27% without unchanged other hemodynamics and renal function. For patients who received 24 hours of treatment ($n = 23$), urine output increased by 130% and net output increased by 156%.

PreCARDIA offers a promising approach for decongestion in ADHF by reducing filling pressure and increasing urine output. Future trials are needed to confirm the clinical utility of this approach in the management of ADHF.

> **Key messages**
> - *Diuretics are often suboptimal for decongestion in ADHF.*
> - *Mechanical approaches to reduce cardiac filling pressure are under trial.*
> - *VENOUS-HF EFS is the first-in-human study with a balloon catheter for decongestion which was found to be efficacious and safe.*

ARTICLE 4

Durability of Benefit after Transcatheter Tricuspid Valve Intervention: Insights from Actigraphy

Stocker TJ, Cohen DJ, Arnold SV, Sommer S, Braun D, Stolz L, et al. Durability of Benefit after Transcatheter Tricuspid Valve Intervention: Insights from Actigraphy.
Eur J Heart Fail. 2022;24(7):1293-301.

Abstract

Aims: A strong association was reported for tricuspid regurgitation (TR) with high mortality, morbidity, and reduced physical capacity. Present study was proposed to examine the long-term impact of transcatheter tricuspid valve intervention (TTVI) by using the method of actigraphy on physical activity.

Methods and results: In this prospective study, 128 heart failure patients with severe TR (median age 79 years, 48% female) included who were scheduled for TTVI. For 1 week before TTVI, patients were equipped with activity tracking devices, and again at 1–6 months and 1 year after TTVI. Here, compared continuous physical activity (CPA), defined as the mean number of steps/day with the New York Heart Association class, quality of life assessments, and 6-minute walk distance (all $p < 0.01$). In 94% of patients TTVI reduced TR to grade ≤2+. At 1 year after TTVI ($p < 0.001$ for both comparisons), median [interquartile range (IQR)] CPA at baseline was 3,108 (1,350–4,959) steps/day, which increased by 31.4% to 3,958 (1,823–5,657) steps/day at 1–6 months, and 4,080 (2,293–6,514) steps/day. In advanced heart failure patients with low baseline activity (baseline CPA < 1,350 steps/day; 1-year CPA increase: +121.3%; $p < 0.001$) the impact of TTVI was significantly higher, when compared to moderate activity patients (baseline CPA 1,350–4,959 steps/day; 1-year CPA increase: +27.5%; $p < 0.01$) or high-activity patients (baseline CPA >4,959 steps/day; 1-year CPA change: +2.6%; $p = 0.39$).

Conclusion: After TTVI, durable improvement of physical activity was demonstrated in 1-week actigraphy. In present study, fragile chronic heart failure patients with very low baseline activity, as determined by actigraphy, meaningfully benefit from transcatheter intervention and should not be excluded from TTVI.

ARTICLE COMMENTARY

Severe tricuspid regurgitation (TR) in the setting of chronic heart failure increases mortality and results in impaired quality of life. Such patients with severe functional disability were previously not considered for any valvular intervention. Several transcatheter tricuspid valve intervention techniques (TTVI) have been developed and have been found to improve quality of life. But, the studies have done so far assessed the patients' physical status by subjective models having inherent limitations. Recently, an objective assessment of daily physical activity by actigraphy has been introduced and found to demonstrate improved physical activity after TTVI. Till now, only postprocedural results were available. So far, no follow-up study was done for physical activity assessment by actigraphy after TTVI in heart failure. This is the first study in the literature.

In a prospective observational study by Stocker et al., 128 eligible patients (median age 79 years, 48% female) with heart failure and significant TR who were considered for TTVI excluding inactive hospitalized patients underwent actigraphy for 1 week in a real-life patient environment. Baseline actigraphy was done with an activity tracking device applied to the wrist 2-6 weeks before TTVI. This device recorded the number of steps and heart rate at home daily between 7:00 AM and 10:00 PM (tracking period). The mean number of steps per day at each tracking period was referred to as continuous physical activity (CPA), which was the study's primary outcome measure. Other outcome measures were steps per day on the day with the highest physical activity (high-performance day) and the lowest activity (low-performance day). The patients were stratified according to their baseline CPA as low activity (<1,350 steps/day), moderate activity (1,350-4,959 steps/day), and high-activity groups (>4,959 steps/day). Clinically significant improvement in CPA was defined as an improvement of 500 steps/day. Another conventional functional assessment was done along with echocardiography at baseline. The first follow-up (FU1) was done at 1-6 months after TTVI and the second follow-up (FU2) was done after 1 year.

Isolated tricuspid edge-to-edge repair was performed in 67%, combined mitral and tricuspid intervention in 31%, and tricuspid annuloplasty in 2%. TR was reduced significantly in 94% of patients. Median CPA increased significantly from 3,108 steps/day at baseline to 3,958 steps/day at FU1, and 4,080 steps/day at FU2. Similarly, at FU2 high-performance days improved by 40.8%, and low-performance days improved by 75.1%. On subgroup analysis, similar results were observed for patients with isolated TTVI. The patients in the low-activity group were more symptomatic, had higher operative risk, and all had TR ≥ grade 3+. This group had the greatest improvement in CPA after TTVI followed by those in the moderate activity group. The patients in the high-activity group showed insignificant changes in CPA. Clinically, significant improvement in CPA was observed in 76% of the low-activity group and 60% in the moderate-activity group. All patients, irrespective of performance groups, had symptomatic improvement, similar survival, heart failure hospitalization, and mortality. Similar results were shown by patients with isolated TTVI. Thus, TTVI improves the quality of life and physical activity in patients with heart failure with significant TR. This study also showed the greatest benefit for patients with low performance at baseline. Hence, all chronic heart failure patients with severe TR may be given the benefit of TTVI if feasible, particularly if they have low physical activity by actigraphy.

> **Key messages**
> - TTVI should be considered in heart failure with severe TR.
> - Actigraphy allows in-home physical activity assessment.

ARTICLE 5

Left Atrial Volume Index and Outcome after Transcatheter Edge-to-edge Valve Repair for Secondary Mitral Regurgitation

Iliadis C, Kalbacher D, Lurz P, Petrescu AM, Orban M, Puscas T, et al. Left atrial volume index and outcome after transcatheter edge-to-edge valve repair for secondary mitral regurgitation.
Eur J Heart Fail. 2022;24(7):1282-92.

Abstract

Aims: In the present study, patients with secondary mitral regurgitation (SMR) undergoing transcatheter edge-to-edge mitral valve repair (TEER) investigation of the role of left atrial volume index (LAVi) were done.

Methods and results: In SMR, patients of a European Multicentre Registry according to baseline LAVi outcomes were evaluated. For all-cause mortality, main analysis was performed; for available patients, residual mitral regurgitation (MR) and the New York Heart Association (NYHA) class improvement were analyzed. Totally 1,074 patients were included with a median LAVi (interquartile range) of 58 mL/m^2 (46–73). Across LAVi quintiles postprocedural reduction of MR grade to ≤2+ was similar, ranging from 91 to 96% ($p = 0.26$). Symptomatic benefit (≥1 NYHA class improvement) also did not differ by LAVi quintiles (61–68% of patients) ($p = 0.66$). In the four upper quintiles in comparison to the bottom quintile (LAVi < 42 mL/m^2) increase of 23–42% risk of mortality was observed. The observed association of the hazard ratio (HR) of mortality 1.35 [95% confidence interval (CI) 1.02–1.78; $p = 0.035$] with a LAVi > 42 mL/m^2, which was attenuated after multivariable adjustment (HR 1.18; 95% CI 0.83–1.67; $p = 0.36$). In multivariable analysis, a significant interaction was noted for MR severity and pulmonary hypertension, with an increased risk of death associated with enlarged LAVi in patients with inframedian effective regurgitant orifice area (HR 1.99; 95% CI 1.06–3.74; $p = 0.032$) and in patients with systolic pulmonary pressure ≤50 mm Hg (HR 1.67; 95% CI 1.02–2.75; $p = 0.042$).

Conclusion: Throughout the whole range of LAVi procedural success and symptomatic benefit were high. The prognostic impact of left atrial enlargement was relevant in patients with less severe SMR and without pulmonary hypertension. These findings emphasize the need to detect patients in the early course of backward congestion to attain good long-term outcomes after TEER.

ARTICLE COMMENTARY

Left ventricular (LV) dysfunction increases left atrial (LA) pressure which results in LA dilatation. This leads to annular dilation causing noncoaptation of mitral leaflets resulting in secondary mitral regurgitation (SMR). SMR adds to LA and LV volume overload which further increases LA size causing increasing severity of mitral regurgitation (MR). This becomes a vicious cycle and can be rightly said that MR begets MR. In recent years, transcatheter edge-to-edge mitral valve repair (TEER) has been developed and studied. However, there are conflicting results. Although an increase in LA size is a predictor of poor outcomes in heart failure (HF), this parameter is not adequately studied in patients with secondary MR undergoing TEER.

Iliadis et al., in their multicenter retrospective study, studied LAVi as a predictor of outcome in patients with SMR undergoing TEER. The primary endpoint was all-cause mortality and the secondary endpoints were HF hospitalization, the combined endpoint of death and HF hospitalization, procedural success defined by postprocedural MR ≤ grade 2+, and improvement in the NYHA class at the last follow-up. The data was collected from the EuroSMR registry including 11 centers across Europe from patients who underwent TEER between 2008 and 2021, and who had preprocedural LAVi values. Patients' characteristics, echocardiographic findings, and all-cause mortality were collected, and patients were stratified based on quantiles of LAVi (≤42, 42–53, 54–62, 63–76, ≥77 mL/m^2).

A total of 1,074 patients (median age 75 years, 66% male) were eligible for the study out of which 92% patients had enlarged LA (LAVi ≥ 34 mL/m^2), while around 70% had severe LA dilatation (LAVi ≥ 48 mL/m^2). The grade of MR significantly improved after TEER ranging from 91 to 96% with no significant difference between different quantiles. The NYHA class significantly improved in all patients with at least one class improvement in 60.9 to 68.3% across LAVi quantiles. 36% of patients died with significantly increased mortality in patients with LAVi > 42 mL/m^2 when compared with those having LAVi ≤ 42 mL/m^2. HF hospitalization occurred in 32% of patients with no significant hazard for patients with LAVi ≥ 42 mL/m^2. Patients with LAVi ≥ 42 mL/m^2 had borderline increased hazard for the combined endpoint of death or HF hospitalization. Significant mortality was observed for patients with LAVi ≥ 42 mL/m^2 who had less severe MR and no pulmonary hypertension even after adjusting for risk predictors of mortality. Interestingly, the trial has shown that patients after undergoing TEER had an improvement in functional class irrespective of LAVi when it is already known that LA size corresponds with symptom burden in these patients independently of LV function. In the study population, only a mild increase in mortality was found for patients with moderate to severe LA enlargement which could be attributed to the success of TEER itself in these patients.

Since TEER has high procedural efficacy and causes significant symptomatic improvement in all patients irrespective of LA size, this should be offered to all patients of heart failure with secondary MR who meets the clinical indication. Although the mortality is higher for higher LA size, these subsets comprise the majority of HF patients and they should not be debarred from the beneficial effects of TEER.

> **Key messages**
> - Patients in HF with secondary MR should be given the benefit of TEER regardless of their LAVi.
> - To alter the natural history of HF with secondary MR, it would be prudent to target those in their early stages.

ARTICLE 6

Transcatheter Repair for Patients with Tricuspid Regurgitation

Sorajja P, Whisenant B, Hamid N, Naik H, Makkar R, Tadros P, et al. Transcatheter Repair for Patients with Tricuspid Regurgitation.
N Engl J Med. 2023;388(20):1833-42.

Abstract

Background: There is an association of a debilitating condition severe tricuspid regurgitation with substantial morbidity and often with poor quality of life. In patients with this disease, decreasing tricuspid regurgitation may reduce symptoms and improve clinical outcomes.

Methods: Present study is a prospective, randomized trial of percutaneous tricuspid transcatheter edge-to-edge repair (TEER) for severe tricuspid regurgitation. In the selected countries, such as the United States, Canada, and Europe patients reported with symptomatic severe tricuspid regurgitation were registered at 65 selected centers and were randomly allocated in a 1:1 ratio to obtain either TEER or medical therapy (control). Around 1-year follow-up of patients, the primary outcome was a hierarchical combination that comprised death resulted from any cause of tricuspid-valve surgery; hospitalization duration for heart failure; and overall, benefit in better quality of life as measured with the Kansas City Cardiomyopathy Questionnaire (KCCQ), with an improvement defined as an increase of at least 15 points in the KCCQ score (range, 0 to 100, with higher scores indicating better quality of life). Also, here they assessed the severity of tricuspid regurgitation and all safety measures.

Results: Overall, 350 patients were enrolled and to each group 175 patients were assigned. The mean age was 78 years of enrolled patients and 54.9% were women. The results for the primary endpoint preferred the TEER group (win ratio: 1.48; 95% CI 1.06–2.13; $p = 0.02$). Between the groups, the incidence of death or tricuspid-valve surgery and the rate of hospitalization for heart failure did not seem to differ. In the TEER group, the KCCQ quality-of-life score changed by a mean (±SD) of 12.3 ± 1.8 points, as compared with 0.6 ± 1.8 points in the control group ($p < 0.001$). 87.0% of the patients in the TEER group and 4.8% in the control group had tricuspid regurgitation of no greater than moderate severity ($p < 0.001$) observed at 30 days. At 30 days, 98.3% of the patients who underwent the procedure were free from major adverse events and TEER was found to be safe.

Conclusion: For patients with severe tricuspid regurgitation tricuspid TEER was safe and reduced the severity of tricuspid regurgitation. Also, an association with an improvement in quality of life was observed.

ARTICLE COMMENTARY

Symptomatic severe tricuspid regurgitation (TR) carries a high degree of morbidity and mortality. However, these patients have multiple comorbidities like previous left-sided heart surgeries, previous mitral or aortic or tricuspid valve surgeries, cardiomyopathies, atrial fibrillation, chronic kidney disease (CKD), and chronic liver disease (CLD) which make them high risk for surgical interventions. Also, surgical treatments carry a high degree of morbidity and mortality. Hence, most of the time the patients were managed with medical management. Hence, the option for less invasive transcatheter tricuspid valve intervention is evolving, which mainly consists of repair system—tricuspid transcatheter edge-to-edge repair (T-TEER), TriClip being the most popular. However, there is no randomized trial data available for the same.

Methodology: Symptomatic severe TR in spite of giving optimal medical management to patients who are at intermediate or greater estimated risk for mortality or morbidity with tricuspid valve surgery. They are found appropriate for TriClip which were registered at 65 predefined centers in the United States, Canada, and Europe and were randomly allocated in a 1:1 ratio to obtain either T-TEER or medical therapy (control). A hierarchical composite that comprised death from any cause/condition or tricuspid-valve surgery; hospitalization duration for heart failure; and an improvement in quality-of-life as measured with the Kansas City Cardiomyopathy Questionnaire (KCCQ) with an improvement defined as an increase of at least 15 points in the KCCQ score at the 1-year follow-up are the primary endpoint.

Results and conclusion: Primary endpoints favored the T-TEER group. This was mainly due to an improvement in quality-of-life, primarily related to the decrease in TR. Between the groups, the frequency of death rates or tricuspid-valve surgery and the repeated hospitalization course for heart failure did not seem to vary greatly. T-TEER has an excellent safety record. It appears that as the therapy evolves, the results might improve further as the risk profile of the patient decreases and procedural expertise increases.

> **Key messages**
> - *This study provides first-ever randomized data for T-TEER.*
> - *T-TEER with Triclip decreases TR thereby leading to improvement in quality of life.*
> - *It can be done with reasonable safety.*
> - *More studies are required to understand the impact on mortality.*

ARTICLE 7

Transcatheter Mitral Valve Replacement or Repair for Secondary Mitral Regurgitation: A Propensity Score-matched Analysis

Ludwig S, Kalbacher D, Ali WB, Weimann J, Adam M, Duncan A, et al. Transcatheter Mitral Valve Replacement or Repair for Secondary Mitral Regurgitation: A Propensity Score-matched Analysis.
Eur J Heart Fail. 2023;25(3):399-410.

Abstract

Aims: For the treatment of secondary mitral regurgitation (SMR), the present study intended to compare outcomes after transcatheter mitral valve replacement (TMVR) and mitral valve transcatheter edge-to-edge repair (M-TEER).

Methods and results: From 2014 to 2022 the CHOICE-MI (CHoice of OptImal transCatheter trEatment for Mitral Insufficiency) registry enrolled a total of 262 patients with SMR treated with TMVR. 1,065 patients with SMR treated with M-TEER enrolled in the Euro SMR registry from 2014 to 2019. For selected 12 demographic, clinical, and echocardiographic parameters propensity score (PS) matching was performed. In the matched cohorts, echocardiographic, functional, and clinical outcomes were compared out to 1 year. TMVR patients 235 [75.5 years (70.0 and 80.0), 60.2% male, EuroSCORE II 6.3% (interquartile range 3.8, 12.4)] were compared to 411 M-TEER patients [76.7 years (70.1 and 80.5), 59.0% male, EuroSCORE II 6.7% (3.9, 12.4)] after PS matching. At 30 days, all-cause mortality was reported to be 6.8% after TMVR and 3.8% after M-TEER ($p = 0.11$), and 25.8% after TMVR, and 18.9% after M-TEER at 1 year ($p = 0.056$). Here, we found no significant differences in mortality after 1 year between both groups in a 30-day landmark analysis (TMVR: 20.4%, M-TEER: 15.8%, and $p = 0.21$). In comparison to M-TEER, TMVR resulted in more effective mitral regurgitation (MR) reduction (residual MR ≤ 1+ at discharge for TMVR vs. M-TEER: 95.8% vs. 68.8%, $p < 0.001$), and superior symptomatic improvement (New York Heart Association class ≤ II at 1 year: 77.8% vs. 64.3%, $p = 0.015$).

Conclusion: In patients with severe SMR, in a PS-matched comparison between TMVR and M-TEER, TMVR was found to be associated with a superior reduction of MR and showed superior symptomatic improvement. Whereas, postprocedural mortality is likely to be higher after TMVR, beyond 30 days no significant differences in mortality were found.

ARTICLE COMMENTARY

Secondary mitral regurgitation (SMR) is associated with increased morbidity and mortality. These patients are at high risk for corrective surgical repair and surgical repair is associated with increased perioperative mortality. Therefore, the majority of these patients are treated with optimal medical therapy. However, when these patients become symptomatic despite optimal medical therapy, they are considered for transcatheter edge-to-edge repair (TEER), the most popular being MitraClip. There are many transcatheter mitral valve replacement (TMVR) systems tried for this subgroup of patients. There are no randomized data available to compare TEER and TMVR for this subgroup of patients. The given article is a propensity score-matched analysis comparing TEER versus TMVR for SMR patients.

The CHOICE-MI registry enrolled 262 patients presented with SMR, treated with TMVR from 2014 to 2022. The EuroSMR registry comprised of 1,065 patients with SMR treated with M-TEER from 2014 to 2019. For 12 demographic, clinical, and echocardiographic parameters, propensity score (PS) matching was done. In the matched cohorts, echocardiographic, functional, and clinical outcomes nearly to 1 year were compared. There was a non-significant trend for increased mortality at 30 days in the TMVR group. However, no significant difference in mortality was found at 1 year between the two groups. TMVR was strongly associated with a superior reduction of MR and superior symptomatic improvement.

> **Key messages**
> - TMVR has the potential to be a therapeutic alternative for patients with SMR.
> - There is a need of randomized data comparing TEER with TMVR.
> - With increasing operator understanding, device evolution, and the alteration to transfemoral devices, a bigger patient population might become eligible and primarily selected for TMVR.

SECTION 11

Digital Technology in Heart Failure

Section Editor: Hetan C Shah

Co-Editors: Prayaag Kinni, Manojit Lodha

ARTICLE 1

Artificial Intelligence in Cardiovascular Medicine: Current Insights and Future Prospects

Haq IU, Chhatwal K, Sanaka K, Xu B. Artificial Intelligence in Cardiovascular Medicine: Current Insights and Future Prospects.
Vasc Health Risk Manag. 2022;18:517-28.

Abstract

The burden on healthcare systems significantly increasing due to cardiovascular disease (CVD). A rapidly evolving transdisciplinary field is artificial intelligence (AI), using mostly machine learning (ML) techniques, to simulate human intuition to offer cost-effective and scalable solutions for better management of CVD. In various facets of cardiovascular medicine, ML algorithms are increasingly being established and applied, including and not limited to heart failure, electrophysiology, valvular heart disease (VHD), and coronary artery disease (CAD). AI algorithms can expand diagnostic capabilities and clinical decision-making through automated cardiac measurements of heart failure. Using ML from diagnostic data occult cardiac disease is increasingly being identified. Enhanced clinical care of VHD patients and CAD achieving because of improved diagnostic and prognostic capabilities using ML algorithms. The development of AI techniques comes with obstacles, the most significant being the need for external validation through conducting multicenter clinical trials.

ARTICLE COMMENTARY

After incidents of kids getting their homework done by an artificial intelligence (AI) based platforms, we surely, as practicing cardiologists have been wondering what AI has brought us. The origins of AI can be traced to Alan Turing who explored the mathematical possibility of AI and apparently, cracked the "Enigma". AI is a rapidly evolving field employing machine learning (ML) techniques, aiming to simulate human intuition, if it has not already done that. ML algorithms are increasingly being developed and applied in heart failure, electrophysiology, and interventional cardiology. AI has brought new horizons at large in all the scientific disciplines and cardiovascular medicine is not exempted from that.

Machine learning includes supervised and unsupervised learning and deep and reinforcement learning. Apparently, ML requires a huge amount of data sets to work and when it comes to healthcare in general, cardiovascular medicine is one subspecialty that has accumulated probably the highest amount of data from the general as well as patient population in recent times. In cardiology, the first application of AI was the development of self-learning neural networks applied to electrocardiography. Since then, AI has come a long way with its applications ranging from its role in the diagnosis and management of heart failure to predicting obstructive coronary artery disease (CAD) in a given patient.

Despite the fact that AI might prove to be a game-changer in upcoming years when it comes to cardiovascular medicines, there are a number of challenges that need to be addressed. With the pace at which AI is growing, it is prudent not to include AI in the upcoming societal guidelines for the management of cardiovascular diseases (CVD). AI requires a huge dataset for any particular function, yet, such databases are largely uncurated. Besides, to feed the AI-based algorithms, data mining is often one of the resorts; however, it is our duty to protect patients' privacy at any cost. Even though there is a possibility that AI-based systems will eventually take over a majority of functions in cardiovascular medicine, the human touch is something that can never be replaced and as gatekeepers of this ever-evolving era, it is our responsibility to look after the nonhindrance of patientcare.

Key messages

- In today's era, there is no option for accepting and evolving with AI-based systems. The involvement of AI in patient care and particularly in cardiovascular medicine is increasing day in and out. From analyzing electrocardiograms to estimating cardiovascular outcomes, AI is going to hold an important place in the management of CVDs.
- Despite the fact that AI is literally taking over healthcare in the near future, there is no substitution for the "humane touch" in clinical medicine. As vigilantes of this concept, we should make sure that the patient remains at the core of healthcare and nothing else.

ARTICLE 2

Electronic Alerts to Improve Heart Failure Therapy in Outpatient Practice a Cluster Randomized Trial

Ghazi L, Yamamoto Y, Riello RJ, Coronel-Moreno C, Martin M, O'Connor KD, et al. Electronic Alerts to Improve Heart Failure Therapy in Outpatient Practice A Cluster Randomized Trial.
J Am Coll Cardiol. 2022;79(22):2203-13.

Abstract

Background: In patients with heart failure with reduced ejection fraction (HFrEF) the use of guideline-directed medical therapy (GDMT) is under-prescribed.

Objectives: Present study aimed to examine whether targeted and tailored electronic health record (EHR) alerts recommending GDMT in eligible HFrEF patients improve GDMT use.

Methods: A realistic, EHR-based, cluster-randomized comparative effectiveness trial was PROMPT-HF (PRagmatic trial Of Messaging to Providers about Treatment of Heart Failure). A total of 100 providers caring for HFrEF patients were randomized to either alert or usual care. Along with patient characteristics, the alert notified providers of individual GDMT recommendations. An increase in the number of GDMT classes prescribed at 30 days postrandomization was the primary outcome of this study. Here, providers' knowledge about guidelines and user experience was surveyed.

Results: In the present study, 1,310 ambulatory patients with HFrEF were enrolled from April to October 2021. Participants' median age was 72 years; comprise 31% female; 18% black; and 32% median left ventricular ejection fraction (LVEF). Beta-blockers were received by 84% of participants, 71% received a renin–angiotensin–aldosterone system (RAAS) inhibitor, 29% received a mineralocorticoid receptor antagonist, and 11% received a sodium-glucose cotransporter-2 (SGLT-2) inhibitor, at baseline. Out of 685 only 176 (26%) participants were in the alert arm versus 117 of 625 (19%) in the usual care arm, thus GDMT class prescription increased by >40% after alert exposure (adjusted relative risk 1.41; 95% CI 1.03–1.93; $p = 0.03$) these are the major primary outcome. The number of patients needed to alert to result in an increase in the addition of GDMT classes was 14. The alert was effective at enabling improved prescription of medical therapy for HF agreed by a total of 79% of alerted providers.

Conclusion: For outpatients with HFrEF, led to significantly higher rates of GDMT at 30 days when equated with usual care, here used a real-time, targeted, and tailored EHR-based alerting system for analysis. In heart failures, this low-cost intervention can be rapidly assimilated into clinical care and may accelerate the adoption of high-value therapies.

ARTICLE COMMENTARY

We, as physicians, have come a long way in terms of providing treatment options for heart failure patients. From the early days of digoxin being invented from a plant as the most effective treatment for heart failure to developing devices for the same, the quality of life of patients suffering from heart failure has increased tremendously. And yet, despite having a guideline directed medical therapy (GDMT) which includes four classes of drugs and then some, is rather under-prescribed in patients with HFrEF.

Ghazi et al. published a cluster of randomized trial to inspect whether targeted and customize electronic health record alerts suggested GDMT in eligible patients presented with heart failure with reduced ejection fraction (HFrEF) shows improved outcomes on GDMT use. This PROMPT-HF (PRagmatic trial Of Messaging to Providers about outpatient Treatment of Heart Failure) study was planned to test the hypothesis that timely informing or upgradations of guidelines about medical treatment of HFrEF especially tailored to the patient's condition would result in higher rates of recommendation of these newer therapies when compared to already known usual care.

All consented physicians were randomized within electronic health record (EHR) system to either the intervention group or the usual care group. This alert educated the healthcare providers/practitioners about the patient's present left ventricular ejection fraction (LVEF) together with the most recent vitals and blood investigations. It also showed the main four pillars of heart failure therapy and showed whether the particular class of medicine was prescribed to the patient or not. Any increase in recommendations for GDMT class was reflected a positive outcome of the study, and a decrease or no change in GDMT was reflected as null findings.

Here, in this present study the primary and secondary outcomes were counted useful when the addition of GDMT class at 30 days and the increase in dose at 30 days respectively. The primary outcome was witnessed in 25.7% of the alert arm and 18.7% of the no alert arm. At baseline, 84% of patients were receiving β blockers, 71% received a renin–angiotensin–aldosterone system (RAAS) inhibitor, 29% received a mineralocorticoid receptor antagonist, and 11% received a sodium-glucose cotransporter-2 (SGLT-2) inhibitor. A total of 79% of alerted providers granted that the alert was beneficial at enabling improved treatment of medical therapy for HF.

To conclude, when compared with already given usual care, a real-time, targeted, and tailored EHR-based notifying system for outpatients with HFrEF referred to significantly showed higher rates of GDMT use at 30 days. However, the most important question is whether such a low-cost and effective intervention can be implemented in developing countries where tertiary-care government hospitals serve the major chunk of population while these facilities are overburdened with patients and the facility of EHR is just taking birth.

Key messages

- The numbers needed to treat (NNT) for aspirin in secondary prevention is 333, while the NNT for mineralocorticoid receptor antagonists (MRAs) in HFrEF is 09. Hence, not prescribing spironolactone to any and all patients eligible for the same with HFrEF is rather grievous, and yet, in the present study, only 29% of patients received MRAs. Hence, if a cost-effective intervention like this can help physicians to prescribe evidence-based GDMT in a better way, they are most welcome.
- In countries like India, where the EHR system is yet in its initial phases, their implementation at large remains a challenge. EHR, as this trial has shown, can be used to provide a better quality of care if used in a substantial way.

ARTICLE 3

Machine Learning-based Prediction of Myocardial Recovery in Patients with Left Ventricular Assist Device Support

Topkara VK, Elias P, Jain R, Sayer G, Burkhoff D, Uriel N. Machine Learning-based Prediction of Myocardial Recovery in Patients with Left Ventricular Assist Device Support.
Circ Heart Fail. 2022;15(1):e008711.

Abstract

Background: In larger numbers of patients supported with left ventricular assist device (LVAD) in *previously published* prospective studies, confirmed that aggressive pharmacological therapy combined with pump speed optimization may result in myocardial recovery. This study was designed to determine the use of machine learning (ML) based model prediction in LVAD patients with myocardial recovery resulting in pump explant.

Methods: In this present study a total of 20,270 adult patients with a durable continuous-flow LVAD in the INTERMACS (Interagency Registry for Mechanically Assisted Circulatory Support) registry were included. For the selection of features associated with LVAD-induced myocardial recovery 98 raw clinical variables were screened by means of the least absolute shrinkage and selection operator. By receiver operating curve and Kaplan–Meier analysis ML models were developed in the training data set (70%) and were considered in the validation of the data set (30%).

Results: Including age, cause of heart failure, psychosocial risk factors, laboratory values, cardiac rate and rhythm, echocardiographic indices, least absolute shrinkage, and selection operator identified 28 distinct clinical features associated with LVAD-induced myocardial recovery.

Machine learning models achieved an area under the receiver operating curve (AUROC) of 0.813–0.824 in the validation data set outperforming logistic regression-based new INTERMACS (Interagency Registry for Mechanically Assisted Circulatory Support) recovery risk score (AUROC of 0.796) and previously established LVAD recovery risk scores [INTERMACS Cardiac Recovery Score (I-CARS) and INTERMACS Recovery Score by Topkara et al. (I-TOPS)] with the AUROC of 0.744 and 0.748 ($p < 0.05$).

A significantly higher incidence of myocardial recovery resulting in LVAD explant in the validation cohort compared with those who were not predicted to recover (18.8% vs. 2.6% at 4 years of pump support) demonstrated in patients who were predicted to recover by ML models.

Conclusion: LVAD patients who may be more likely to respond to myocardial recovery protocols in these subsets of patients, ML can become a valuable tool for identification.

ARTICLE COMMENTARY

Device-based remote monitoring of hemodynamic parameters in heart failure (HF) patients is an exciting facet of artificial intelligence and remote monitoring technology. The use of intrathoracic impedance as a unique monitoring parameter to guide the management is limited by the late onset of pulmonary congestion. Rather, using hemodynamic monitoring allows detection of an early increase in intracardiac or pulmonary artery pressures that represent an early sign of worsening HF and facilitates a prompt and targeted therapeutic response—*"further studies in this regard boosted by probably simultaneous invasive catheterization-based data to boost their accuracy will be something to look forward in the future"*.

ARTICLE 4

Device-based Remote Monitoring Strategies for Congestion-guided Management of Patients with Heart Failure: A Systematic Review and Meta-analysis

Zito A, Princi G, Romiti GF, Galli M, Basili S, Liuzzo G, et al. Device-based Remote Monitoring Strategies for Congestion-guided Management of Patients with Heart Failure: A Systematic Review and Meta-analysis.
Eur J Heart Fail. 2022;24(12):2333-41.

Abstract

Aims: Devices monitoring preclinical congestion markers, of worsening heart failure (HF) may support the management of HF patients. This study aimed to evaluate effectiveness of congestion-guided HF management according to device-based remote monitoring strategies with standard therapy.

Objectives: On PubMed, Embase, and CENTRAL databases a comprehensive literature research for randomized controlled trials (RCTs) for comparing device-based remote monitoring strategies for congestion-guided HF management versus standard therapy was performed. Using the Poisson regression model with random study effects incidence rate ratios (IRRs) and associated 95% confidence intervals (CIs) were calculated. The primary findings were a combination of all-cause death and HF hospitalizations. Secondary endpoints involved the individual components of the primary outcome. A total number of 4347 patients from eight RCTs were included in the present study. According to the type of parameters monitored. Hemodynamic-guided strategy (4 trials, 2,224 patients, and 12-month follow-up) reduced the risk of the primary composite outcome (IRR 0.79; 95% CI 0.70–0.89) and HF hospitalizations (IRR 0.76; 95% CI 0.67–0.86), without any significant impact on all-cause death (IRR 0.93; 95% CI 0.72–1.21) when compared with standard therapy. In comparison, significant benefits were not provided by impedance-guided strategy (4 trials, 2,123 patients, and 19-month follow-up).

Conclusion: Author found a significant association of hemodynamic-guided HF management with better clinical outcomes when compared to standard clinical care.

ARTICLE COMMENTARY

Artificial intelligence (AI) and machine learning (ML) are good tools to predict early decompensation allowing simplification of the treatment of heart failure (HF). It is not an overstatement to consider a strong potential for false discoveries and biases due to "GIGO" (Garbage in Garbage out) creeping in while using them for predictive analysis. This was amply demonstrated by the failure of the much-hyped IBM Watson program. We believe however that this error can be minimized by the concerned medical team by keeping in mind the clinical relevance of the predictors generated by ML-models during the algorithm training and development, thus allowing the wider use of this emerging technology.

ARTICLE 5

Applications of Machine Learning in Cardiology

Seetharam K, Balla S, Bianco C, Cheung J, Pachulski R, Asti D, et al. Applications of Machine Learning in Cardiology. *Cardiol Ther. 2022;11:355-68.*

Abstract

In this phase of digital era, AI is gaining attention in the commercial industry and the technology sector. These developments have strong impact on the healthcare sector, particularly in the clinical field of cardiology, where machine learning (ML) algorithms are making significant advances in various sub-specialities of cardiology, which will ultimately improve patient care and push the field toward precision medicine. This review article examines the development of ML in the fields of cardiovascular imaging, cardiovascular electrocardiography, cardiac failure, and Interventional cardiology.

ARTICLE COMMENTARY

Machine learning (ML) is used to develop models for predicting mortality and heart failure (HF) hospitalization for outpatients with heart failure with preserved ejection fraction (HFpEF) in the TOPCAT (Treatment of Preserved Cardiac Function Heart Failure with an Aldosterone Antagonist) trial. Using logistic regression (LR) with a forward selection of variables using random forest (RF), gradient boosting, and support vector machine (SVM) to train models for assessing risks of mortality and HF hospitalization through 3 years of follow-up, they concluded RF to be the best-performing model with a mean C-statistic of 0.72 for predicting mortality (Brier score: 0.17), and 0.76 for HF hospitalization (Brier score: 0.19). Blood urea nitrogen (BUN) levels, body mass index (BMI), and the Kansas City Cardiomyopathy Questionnaire (KCCQ) scores were shown to be strongly associated with mortality. Similar pioneering studies done by Wang et al., Lancaster et al. and Sanchez-Martinez et al. studied the application of ML to generate predictive models of HF in reduced left ventricular ejection fraction (LVEF) (Wang et al.), and preserved LVEF (the latter two) in patients with HF with the good predictive ability and better accuracy than LR-derived models alone.

With smartphones and mobile apps becoming a part of our daily lifestyle, the concept of a "smart clinic" employing a variety of miniaturized devices including but not limited to POCUS (point-of-care ultrasound), mobile and transmission-enabled ECG and ECHO readers, and amalgamating data from wearable devices like the Fitbit and other smartphone applications may be able to provide continuous data thus enabling the provision of precision medicine at the point of care services in heart failure (HF) cohorts of both reduced and preserved ejection fractions.

ARTICLE 6

Effects of Remote Hemodynamic-guided Heart Failure Management in Patients with Different Subtypes of Pulmonary Hypertension: Insights from the MEMS-HF Study

Assmus B, Angermann CE, Alkhlout B, Asselbergs FW, Schnupp S, Brugts JJ, et al. Effects of remote haemodynamic-guided heart failure management in patients with different subtypes of pulmonary hypertension: insights from the MEMS-HF study.
Eur J Heart Fail. 2022;24(12):2320-30.

Abstract

Aim: During the previous 12 months the CardioMEMS European Monitoring Study for Heart Failure (MEMS-HF) inspected the safety and efficacy of pulmonary artery pressure (PAP)-leading the way for remote patient management (RPM) in New York Heart Association (NYHA) with at least one heart failure hospitalization (HFH) of class III outpatients. Here, they investigated prespecified subgroup analysis to know if RPM effects depended on the presence and subtype of pulmonary hypertension (PH).

Methods and results: Swan–Ganz catheter tracings attained during sensor implant were available for offline manual analysis jointly performed by two experts for 106/234 MEMS-HF participants. According to current PH definitions, all patients were classified into subgroups. Isolated postcapillary PH (IpcPH) and combined post- and precapillary PH (CpcPH) were present in 38 and 36 patients, respectively, whereas 31 patients had no PH. Among patients with PH, pulmonary vascular resistance was higher ($p = 0.029$) and pulmonary artery compliance was lower ($p = 0.003$) in patients with CpcPH and clinical characteristics were comparable between subgroups. All PAPs declined in IpcPH and CpcPH subgroups (all $p < 0.05$), whereas only mean and diastolic PAP decreased in patients without PH (both $p < 0.05$) during 12 months of PAP-guided RPM. Improvements in post- versus preimplant HFH rates were similar in CpcPH [0.639 events/patient-year; hazard ratio (HR) 0.37] and IpcPH (0.72 events/patient-year; HR 0.45) patients. Members without PH are the most benefited ones (0.26 events/patient-year; HR 0.17, $p = 0.04$ vs. IpcPH/CpcPH patients). In all subgroups, quality of life and the New York Heart Association (NYHA) class significantly improved.

Conclusion: Irrespective of the presence or subtype of PH at baseline outpatients with NYHA class III symptoms with at least one HFH during 1-year preimplant significantly benefited from PAP-guided RPM during postimplant follow-up.

ARTICLE COMMENTARY

■ INFERENCE

Patients with heart failure (HF) and New York Heart Association (NYHA) class III symptoms with at least 1 heart failure hospitalization (HFH) in the previous 1 year benefited substantially from pulmonary artery pressure (PAP)-guided remote patient management (RPM) during postsensor implant follow-up. The benefit was consistency irrespective of the presence or subtype of pulmonary hypertension (PH) at baseline.

■ PERSPECTIVE

Recurrences of HF, even after guideline-directed medical therapy and device are most frustrating to the clinician, portend a poor prognosis, and lack proven therapy. RPM is an important tool in advanced HF management by shifting from "reactive" treatment for congestion to "preemptive" and individualized medical intervention, utilizing the actionable signal.

■ STUDY QUESTION

Whether the benefit of RPM in NYHA class III outpatients with HF is affected by the presence and subtype of PH.

This is a prespecified subgroup analysis of the MEMS-HF study, which was a multicenter, prospective, post-marketing study, that characterize the use of the CardioMEMS™ HF sensor system (Abbott, Sylmar, CA, USA). The mother study included 31 centers and 234 patients with NYHA class III HF symptoms over the previous 30 days along with a history of one HFH over the previous 12 months. The subgroup included 106 amongst the MEMS-HF participants, who required right heart catheterization (RHC), done during sensor implant. RHC-derived PAP and pulmonary artery wedge pressure (PAWP) tracings were then reviewed and manually analyzed. Health-related quality of life (HRQOL) was assessed at baseline, and after 6 and 12 months using the Kansas City Cardiomyopathy Questionnaire (KCCQ).

Those 106 sub-study participants were divided into 2 groups: (1) 75 patients suffered from PH (mean PAP ≥ 25 mm Hg) (2) 31 patients did not have any PH. In the first group, 38 patients had isolated post-capillary PH (IpcPH) and 36 patients had combined post- and pre-capillary PH (CpcPH), whereas PH in 1 patient could not be classified. During 12 months of pulmonary artery pressure (PAP)-guided RMP, PAP was reduced in both groups. The decline was maximal in patients with IpcPH ($p < 0.008$), lesser extent in patients with CpcPH ($p = 0.008$), and lowest in patients with no PH ($p = 0.086$). The decline of NT-proBNP after sensor implant was found in all groups and most pronounced in patients with CpcPH. Improvement in QOL was achieved substantially in all patients, irrespective of PH. Similarly, irrespective of PH, all patients were reset from NYHA class III to class II or class I. There was a substantial reduction in post-implant HFH rate in all groups. Interestingly, the reduction was highest in patients without PH (0.26 events/patient-year; HR 0.17, $p = 0.04$) and modest both in patients with IpcPH (0.72 events/patient-year; HR 0.45) and patients with CpcPH (0.63 events/patient-year; HR 0.37).

ARTICLE 7

Longer-term Effects of Remote Patient Management Following Hospital Discharge after Acute Systolic Heart Failure: The Randomized E-INH Trial

Angermann CE, Sehner S, Faller H, Güder G, Morbach C, Frantz S, et al. Longer-Term Effects of Remote Patient Management Following Hospital Discharge After Acute Systolic Heart Failure: The Randomized E-INH Trial. *JACC Heart Fail. 2023;11(2):191-206.*

Abstract

Background: The randomized trial INH (Interdisciplinary Network Heart Failure) ($N = 715$) stated that 6 months' remote patient management (RPM) (HeartNetCare-HF) not diminishes the primary outcome (time to all-cause death/rehospitalization) versus usual care (UC) in discharged patients for acute heart failure after admission, but suggested the better quality of life and lower mortality in the RPM group.

Objectives: The Extended (E)-INH trial examined the effects of 18 months HeartNetCare-HF in an expanded population on the same primary outcome ($N = 1,022$) and after RPM termination, followed by survivors up to 60 months (primary outcome events) or up to 120 months (mortality).

Methods: All suitable patients aged ≥18 years, for acute heart failure, were hospitalized, and with predischarge ejection fraction ≤40% randomized to RPM (RPM + UC; $n = 509$) or control (UC; $n = 513$). Every 6 months during RPM, follow-up visits were scheduled, and then at 36, 60, and 120 months.

Results: No difference was noticed for primary outcome between groups at 18 months [60.7% (95% CI 56.5–65.0%) vs. 61.2% (95% CI 57.0–65.4%)] or 60 months [78.1% (95% CI 74.4–81.6%) vs. 82.8% (95% CI 79.5–86.0%)]. Although, at 60 and 120 months, all-cause mortality was found to be lower in patients who previously undergoing RPM [41.1% (95% CI 37.0–45.5%) vs. 47.4%

(95% CI 43.2–51.8%); p = 0.040 and 64.0% (95% CI 59.8–68.2%) vs. 69.6% (95% CI 65.6–73.5%); p = 0.019]. Health-related quality of life was better in patients, at all visits, exposed to HeartNetCare-HF versus UC.

Conclusion: Even though, 18 months' HeartNetCare-HF did not show a significant reduction in the primary outcome of death or rehospitalization at 60 months, observed lesser 120-month mortality in patients previously undertaking HeartNetCare-HF suggested valuable longer-term effects, while the possibility of a chance finding remains unclear.

ARTICLE COMMENTARY

■ INFERENCE

Patients with heart failure with reduced ejection fraction (HFrEF) who were admitted with acute systolic heart failure benefited significantly in the long term after discharge if they are put on remote patient management (RPM). Both all-cause mortality and cardiovascular mortality were reduced in the RPM arm even 102 months after discontinuing RPM. There was also a significant improvement in the quality of life. This may partially be due to the patient's active involvement and shared responsibility in taking care of his own health and the results take time to materialize.

■ PERSPECTIVE

Despite recent advances in guideline-directed medical therapy (GDMT) in the management of HFrEF, there remains substantial mortality and risk of recurrent hospitalization. There is a huge economic burden associated with this. RPM is an important tool in advanced HF management by shifting from "reactive" treatment for congestion to "preemptive" and individualized medical intervention. RPM can be a significant tool in a country like India where a significant majority resides in rural areas, where access to healthcare providers is limited, but access to smartphones and the internet is widely available. With the help of technology and a system in place, a large number of patients can benefit.

■ STUDY QUESTION

The long-term impact of RPM, including mortality reduction and recurrent hospitalization in patients admitted with HFrEF, after hospital discharge on extended follow-up up to 10 years.

This was a prospective, randomized, parallel-group, controlled, a multicentric study funded by the Federal Ministry of Education and Research, Berlin, Germany. The study included all patients (>18 years) hospitalized with HFrEF (EF < 40%) without new-onset structural heart disease and mental illness. Patients were randomized in 1:1 fashion in 2 arms (RPM + Usual Care vs. UC). About 1,022 eligible patients were followed up every 6 months during RPM and then at 36, 60 and 120 months. RPM is structured telephone monitoring and 19-items standardizes questionnaires including medical adherence and side effects.

A total of 1,543 patients were screened and 1,032 eligible patients were randomized in a 1:1 fashion in RPM + UC versus UC using computerized stratification based on Age (<70/>70 years), sex, and type of post-discharge care (general practitioner or cardiologist). Primary outcome (time to the first event of the composite of all causes death or hospitalization) did not differ between the groups at 18 months or 60 months.

But all-cause mortality was lower in the RPM arm at 60 months and 120 months [41.1% (95% CI 37.0–45.5%) vs. 47.4% (95% CI 43.2–51.8%); p –0.040 and 64.0% (95% CI 59.8–68.2%) vs. 69.6% (95% CI 65.6–73.5%]; p –0.019). Cardiovascular mortality was also lower in the RPM arm at the end of 10 years follow-up. At all visits, health-related quality of life adjudged by KCCQ score was better in patients exposed to RPM vis-a-vis usual care group. Throughout the study period, patients included in the RPM group must maintain a lower heart rate and improved NYHA functional class.

SECTION 12

Miscellaneous

Section Editor: Tripti Deb

Co-Editors: Sharad Chandra, Suman Jatain

ARTICLE 1

Nutrition Assessment and Dietary Interventions in Heart Failure JACC Review Topic of the Week

Driggin E, Cohen LP, Gallagher D, Karmally W, Maddox T, Hummel SL, et al. Nutrition Assessment and Dietary Interventions in Heart Failure: JACC Review Topic of the Week.
J Am Coll Cardiol. 2022;79(16):1623-35.

Abstract

Substantial heart failure (HF) guidelines lack specific nutrition recommendations, regardless of the high prevalence of nutrition disorders in patients with HF. In view of fact that standardized definitions and assessment tools to quantify nutritional status are less well-documented, nutrition disorders are often missed in HF patients. In addition, in this population, a comprehensive range of dietary interventions and overall dietary patterns analyzed. There was a conflict in the resulting evidence, making it challenging to govern which strategies are the most beneficial. In present study, they reviewed mostly available nutritional status assessment tools for patients with HF. However, they appraised the current evidence for dietary interventions in HF, comprising sodium restriction, obesity, malnutrition, dietary patterns, and specific macronutrient and micronutrient supplementation. Likewise, here in this document discussed the major challenges and feasibility associated with the implementation of multimodal nutrition interventions and outline the potential explanations to facilitate addressing nutrition in patients with HF.

ARTICLE COMMENTARY

The article aims to provide a comprehensive review of the role of diet in heart failure (HF), including the impact of macronutrients, micronutrients, and dietary patterns on HF outcomes. The article also appraises the current evidence for dietary interventions in HF, including sodium restriction, obesity, malnutrition, and dietary patterns. The study involves reviewing available nutritional status assessment tools for patients with HF and appraising the current evidence for dietary interventions in HF **(Fig. 1)**.

The wide range of prevalence estimates (15-90%) underscores the need for

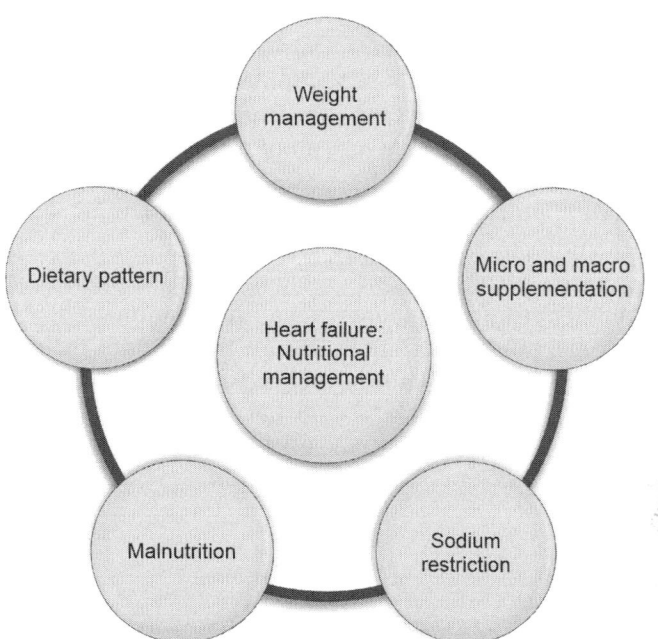

FIG. 1: Nutritional management of heart failure.

standardized definitions and assessment tools to accurately identify malnutrition in patients with HF.

There is evidence of an "obesity paradox" in HF, where patients with higher body mass index (BMI) have better survival rates than those with lower BMI. Patients with morbid obesity (BMI > 40 kg/m^2) do not have the same survival advantage as their obese counterparts.

Malnutrition is an important poor prognostic factor for chronic HF and advanced HF. Nutritional screening and assessment tools can be used to predict all-cause mortality in patients with HF.

Certain dietary patterns were associated with the development of heart failure with reduced ejection fraction (HFrEF) but not heart failure with preserved ejection fraction (HFpEF). Adherence to a Mediterranean-style diet is associated with reduced risk of HF. The DASH (Dietary Approaches to Stop Hypertension) diet may have benefits in secondary prevention of HF.

Current guidelines recommend that patients with symptomatic HF should restrict sodium intake to 2–3 g/day or less. However, the evidence supporting the restriction of dietary sodium intake in HF patients is unclear and that patient adherence to dietary sodium restriction is poor.

Micronutrient deficiencies in HF are the mainly cause because of poor dietary intake along with increased urinary output with more diuretic agents. Till date the only treatment is iron supplementation with resulted from iron deficiency. While it was observed that oral iron supplementation is not able to show better clinical outcomes, as given intravenous iron has presented much advantage for improved functional capacity and better quality of life. Generally, it is expected that most of the known micronutrient deficiencies can be treated by a nutritious diet plans.

Supplementation with unsaturated fatty acids (UFAs) has been shown to improve cardiorespiratory fitness (CRF) in patients presented with HFpEF and with other condition like obesity studies in a single-arm pilot study. Though, a current published meta-analysis verified a higher risk for incident atrial fibrillation with n-3 polyunsaturated fatty acid (PUFA) in patients with well-known traditional factors or who are at high risk for cardiovascular disease. Most benefits in CRF among patients with sarcopenia and/or cardiac cachexia seen, when given supplementation with amino acids and/or protein. This treatment revealed to be modest although till date this is not routinely recommended.

To conclude despite the high prevalence of nutrition disorders in patients with HF, major HF guidelines lack specific nutrition recommendations. Population-based education is essential to improve nutritional related morbidity. Further research is needed to better understand the optimal dietary approach for patients with HF.

ARTICLE 2

Spirituality in Patients with Heart Failure

Tobin RS, Cosiano MF, O'Connor CM, Fiuzat M, Granger BB, Rogers JG, et al. Spirituality in Patients With Heart Failure. *JACC Heart Fail. 2022;10(4):217-26.*

Abstract

A core domain of gentle care, dynamic, and multidimensional aspect of oneself for which one aspect is of finding meaning and purpose is defined as spirituality. Presently with more developed treatment options in heart failure (HF), patients are living longer, putting further importance on quality of life (QOL) and on the role of palliative care principles in their care. Till date significant data published to describe the role of spirituality in cancer patients but still limited number of studies in HF. In this review article, here explored the current information about spirituality in HF patients; also, define associations between spirituality, QOL, and HF outcomes; and recommend clinical applications and future directions concerning spiritual care in present population. Previously published studies indicated that to improve QOL caregiver support, and patient an outcome comprising rehospitalization and mortality, spirituality serves as a potential target for palliative care interventions. Present study revealed that to identify HF patients at risk for spiritual distress, the development of a spirituality-screening tool, similar to the Patient Health Questionnaire-2, is used to screen for depression may be helpful in designing the future management strategies. By members of study group, novel tools are soon to be validated. Less is known about the spirituality in HF compared with other patient populations, so further controlled trials and uniform measures of spirituality are needed to better understand its impact.

ARTICLE COMMENTARY

The study on "Spirituality in Patients with Heart Failure" emphasizes the importance of addressing the spiritual needs of patients with heart failure (HF). The findings suggest that spirituality is prevalent among patients with HF, and there are unaddressed spiritual needs within this population. Patients with HF often experience poor quality of life (QOL), high levels of anxiety and depression, and spirituality has been found to have a positive impact on these aspects.

The "Report of the Consensus Conference" defines spirituality as an essential dimension of palliative care that includes meaning, connectedness to spirituality as an aspect of humanity, and the search for the significant or sacred.[1]

The study highlights that spirituality can improve the QOL for patients with heart failure **(Fig. 2)**. It suggests that spirituality should be considered as a potential target for palliative care interventions to enhance patient-centered care and clinical outcomes. Research has shown that spirituality is instrumental in improving the QOL of patients with HF globally.

In addition, patients with advanced HF who receive advanced therapies such as left ventricular assist devices (LVADs) and cardiac transplants face unique physical and emotional challenges. It is noted that spirituality is one of the domains of QOL in these patients, and even nonreligious participants reported experiences related to meaning, peace, and purpose. Therefore, spirituality is considered important in addressing the specific needs of patients receiving advanced therapies.

Patients with HF commonly experience poor QOL with high levels of anxiety and depression. Depression is present in approximately 20–50% of patients with HF, and with higher levels of depression associated with increased morbidity and mortality. Anxiety has been identified at similar rates as depression in patients with HF. The study suggests that spirituality could serve as a support tool for caregivers and that they

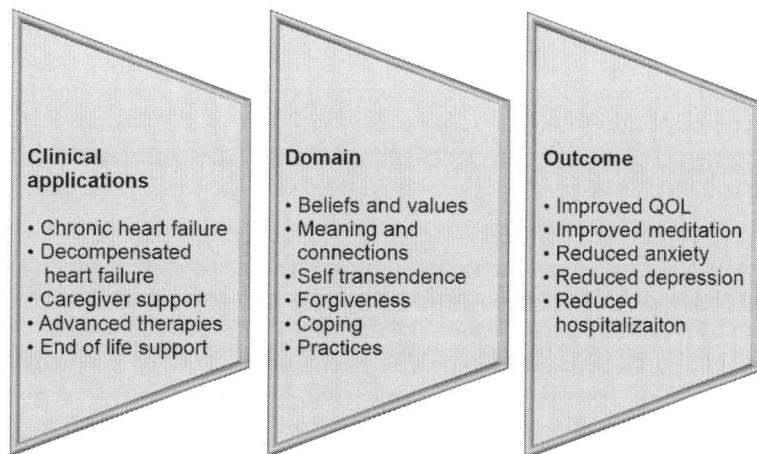

FIG. 2: Heart failure: Clinical applications, domain, and outcome.
(QOL: quality of life)

could benefit from targeted spiritual interventions. However, further research is needed to explore the relationship between spirituality and the well-being of caregivers in this context.

To address the spiritual needs of patients with HF, the study proposes the development of a spirituality screening tool that can identify patients at risk of spiritual distress and those who would benefit from spirituality-based interventions. The goal is to have a concise questionnaire that can be easily completed by patients as part of their previsit paperwork.

Overall, the study highlights the limited research on spirituality in patients with HF and calls for further investigations to better understand the role of spirituality in improving QOL and outcomes in this patient population. It emphasizes the need for spirituality to be incorporated into the care of patients with HF, and for healthcare providers to consider their spiritual needs in treatment planning.

ARTICLE 3

Intravenous Ferric Derisomaltose in Patients with Heart Failure and Iron Deficiency in the UK (IRONMAN): An Investigator-initiated, Prospective, Randomized, Open-label, Blinded-endpoint Trial

Kalra PR, Cleland JGF, Petrie MC, Thomson EA, Kalra PA, Squire IB, et al.; IRONMAN Study Group. Intravenous Ferric Derisomaltose in Patients with Heart Failure and Iron Deficiency in the UK (IRONMAN): An Investigator-initiated, Prospective, Randomised, Open-Label, Blinded-endpoint Trial. *Lancet. 2022;400(10369):2199-209.*

Abstract

Background: Intravenous ferric carboxymaltose administration improves quality of life and exercise capacity in the short-term for patients with heart failure (HF), reduced left ventricular ejection fraction and iron deficiency, and reduces hospital admissions for HF up to 1 year. Present study intended to assess the longer-term effects of intravenous ferric derisomaltose on cardiovascular events in HF patients.

Methods: This was a prospective, randomized, open-label, blinded-endpoint trial named as IRONMAN completed in the UK at 70 hospitals. Eligible patients who were aged 18 years or older presented with HF (left ventricular ejection fraction ≤45%) and transferrin saturation <20% or serum ferritin <100 μg/L. Using a web-based system, participants were randomly assigned (1:1) to intravenous ferric derisomaltose or usual care, followed by recruitment context and trial site. This was an open-label trial with masked resolution of the outcomes. By considering patient's bodyweight intravenous ferric derisomaltose dose and hemoglobin concentration was determined. Recurrent hospital admissions for HF and cardiovascular death are the primary endpoints assessed in all validly randomly assigned patients. In all patients assigned to ferric derisomaltose who received at least one infusion and all patients' assigned to usual care safety was assessed. On September 30, 2020, a coronavirus disease 2019 (COVID-19) sensitivity analysis censoring follow-up was prespecified. IRONMAN is registered with ClinicalTrials.gov, NCT02642562.

Findings: Patients were screened for eligibility from August 25, 2016 to October 15, 2021, 1,869, 1,137 patients were randomly allocated to receive intravenous ferric derisomaltose ($n = 569$) or usual care ($n = 568$). 2.7 years was median follow-up time (IQR 1.8–3.6). In the ferric derisomaltose group, 336 primary endpoints (22.4 per 100 patient-years) occurred and 411 (27.5 per 100 patient-years) occurred in the usual care group [rate ratio (RR) 0·82 (95% CI 0.66–1.02); $p = 0.070$]. 210 primary endpoints (22.3 per 100 patient-years) occurred in the ferric derisomaltose group compared with 280 (29.3 per 100 patient-years) in the usual care group [RR 0.76 (95% CI 0.58–1.00); $p = 0·047$], in the COVID-19 analysis. Not observed between-group differences in deaths or hospitalizations due to infections. In the ferric derisomaltose group, fewer patients had shown serious cardiac adverse events [200 (36%)] than in the usual care group [243 (43%)]; difference –7.00% (95% CI –12.69 to –1.32); $p = 0.016$.

Interpretation: Intravenous ferric derisomaltose administration was associated with a lower risk of hospital admissions for HF and cardiovascular death, and included a broad range of patients with HF reduced left ventricular ejection fraction and iron deficiency. In present studied population, these facts support the benefit of iron repletion.

ARTICLE COMMENTARY

Clinical trials showing the effectiveness of intravenous ferric carboxymaltose (FCM) treatment in symptomatic patients with stable chronic heart failure (CHF) [left ventricular ejection fraction (LVEF) 45%] and iron deficiency include FAIR-HF,[2] CONFIRM-HF,[3] and EFFECT-HF,[4] as well as meta-analyses of randomized clinical trials.[5] The future application of a novel intravenous (IV) iron therapy formulation for HF may be influenced by a recent study. IRONMAN[6] (intravenous ferric derisomaltose in patients with HF and iron deficiency in the UK) was the first large-scale, randomized, prospective study to examine the safety and long-term effects of IV ferric derisomaltose in 1,137 adult patients with new or established symptoms of HF, evidence of iron deficiency (serum ferritin 100 g/L or transferrin saturation 20%), and a left ventricular ejection fraction (LVEF) of 45% versus standard care groups. At a median follow-up of 2.7 years, IV ferric derisomaltose reduced the incidence of the primary endpoint of recurrent hospital admissions for HF and cardiovascular (CV) death by 18% compared to standard care (RR 082; 95% CI 0.66–1.0; $p = 0.070$) and missed statistical significance by a small margin. However, the prespecified COVID-19 sensitivity analysis, which included 91% of the study population and negated the possibility of treatment effect diminution due to reduced redosing during the COVID pandemic, revealed a marginal but significant 24% reduction in the primary endpoint ($p = 0.047$), primarily driven by a decrease in HFH, while CV mortality remained unchanged (24% vs. 21%; $p = 0.23$).

This study adds to the accumulating body of consistent evidence that IV iron reduces HFH in iron-deficient patients.[1-4] In addition to the difference in iron formulation, IRONMAN differs from previous trials of iron in HF in that extended follow-up provides assurance of ferric derisomaltose's long-term safety. In addition, it was an open-label study, unlike previous studies of ferric carboxymaltose, with quality of life and exercise capacity as endpoints, necessitating double blinding. IRONMAN defined iron deficiency as a TSAT 20% or ferritin 100 g/L, whereas most previous trials, including the recently concluded AFFIRM-AHF, defined it as ferritin 100 g/L or ferritin 100–299 g/L with a TSAT 20%.[2,3] In the absence of diagnostic criteria for iron deficiency in HF, the current criteria are founded on expert opinion derived from patients with chronic kidney disease. As a result, a substantial number of individuals who are not truly iron-deficient at the cellular level in the cardiovascular system may be misclassified, which can influence trial results.

Another important aspect is that only 3% of participants in this trial were on sodium-glucose cotransporter-2 inhibitors (SGLT-2Is). Dapagliflozin has been shown to increase hematocrit and erythropoiesis, with corresponding reductions in circulating ferritin and TSAT levels due to the alleviation of inflammation-mediated changes in iron homeostasis. However, these results do not suggest a depletion of intracellular iron stores, which could render treatment with intravenous iron unnecessary. Any potential synergistic or antagonistic interactions between contemporary guideline-directed medical therapy (GDMT) (particularly SGLT-2Is) and intravenous iron are not known, and to fill this gap, we need further study.

In IRONMAN, 17% of patients in the control group received oral iron supplementation, which possibly diluted any potential beneficial effect of IV iron in the treatment group. Subdividing the control arm into oral and intravenous iron therapy would have better permitted a comparison of the two, thereby enhancing the trial's value.

Intravenous ferric derisomaltose is added to the arsenal for patients of HF with reduced ejection fraction (HFrEF) or mildly reduced ejection fraction (HFmrEF) LVEF, and iron deficiency, owing to its outstanding tolerability and long-term safety data from the IRONMAN trial. Although additional trials are necessary to draw a conclusion regarding the primary endpoint of HFH and CV mortality, the reduction of CV mortality remains an unattainable objective. The ongoing trial, HEART-FID, with three times the sample size of IRONMAN, will likely help to resolve any unanswered questions regarding iron supplementation and will presumably corroborate the findings of earlier studies.

ARTICLE 4

Impact of Ischemic Etiology on the Efficacy of Intravenous Ferric Carboxymaltose in Patients with Iron Deficiency and Acute Heart Failure: Insights from the AFFIRM-AHF Trial

Metra M, Jankowska EA, Pagnesi M, Anker SD, Butler J, Dorigotti F, et al.; AFFIRM-AHF Investigators. Impact of ischaemic aetiology on the efficacy of intravenous ferric carboxymaltose in patients with iron deficiency and acute heart failure: insights from the AFFIRM-AHF trial.
Eur J Heart Fail. 2022;24(10):1928-39.
Erratum in: *Eur J Heart Fail. 2023;25(3):444.*

Abstract

Aims: Intravenous ferric carboxymaltose (FCM) reduced the heart failure (HF) hospitalizations in AFFIRM-AHF and improved quality of life versus placebo in iron-deficient patients stabilized after an acute HF episode. This study is planned to explain the effects of FCM versus placebo in patients with ischemic and nonischemic HF etiology.

Methods and results: In this present study, 1,082 patients from AFFIRM-AHF were included: 590 reported with ischemic HF (commonly known as investigator-reported ischemic HF etiology and/or prior acute myocardial infarction and/or prior coronary revascularization) and 492 reported with nonischemic HF. In the ischemic HF subgroup, the prevalence of male sex, comorbidities, and history of HF were higher in comparison to nonischemic HF subgroup. For the primary composite outcome annualized event rates of total HF hospitalizations and cardiovascular death with FCM versus placebo were 65.3 versus 100.6 per 100 patient-years in the ischemic HF subgroup [rate ratio (RR) 0.65; 95% confidence interval (CI) 0.47–0.89; $p = 0.007$] and in the nonischemic HF subgroup 58.3 versus 52.5 (RR 1.11; 95% CI 0.75–1.66; $p = 0.60$) (p interaction = 0.039). For the secondary outcome of total HF hospitalizations, an interaction between HF etiology and treatment effect was also observed (p interaction = 0.038). Within each subgroup, using the 12-item Kansas City Cardiomyopathy Questionnaire, a nominal increase in quality of life assessed and observed with FCM versus placebo.

Conclusion: In ischemic patients presented with heart failure, it was observed that hospitalizations and cardiovascular deaths noted at a higher rate on comparison to those who presented with nonischemic HF; also, it was noted that this was reduced by FCM versus placebo only in ischemic patients. Further, research studies are essential to exactly assess the role of etiology in FCM efficacy.

ARTICLE COMMENTARY

Iron deficiency is a common condition observed in approximately 80% of patients with acute heart failure (AHF) and 50% of patients with chronic heart failure (CHF) and is independent of the presence of anemia.[7,8] Clinical trials FAIR-HF,[2] CONFIRM-HF,[3] and EFFECT-HF,[4] as well as meta-analyses of randomized clinical trials[9] provide evidence for the use of IV iron in symptomatic patients with stable CHF (LVEF 45%) and iron deficiency. The unexplored area of the effectiveness and safety of intravenous ferric carboxymaltose (FCM) therapy in stabilized acute HF patients was investigated in the AFFIRM-AHF[10] (a Randomized, Double-blind Placebo-Controlled Trial Comparing the Effect of Intravenous FCM on Hospitalizations and Mortality in Iron Deficient Subjects Admitted with Acute Heart Failure) trial. Patients hospitalized with AHF and an elevated natriuretic peptide level, treated with at least 40 mg of furosemide or equivalent IV diuretics, LVEF 50%, and concurrent iron deficiency were included in the study. A prespecified pre-COVID-19 sensitivity analysis with follow-up censored for the epidemic revealed a significant decrease in the primary outcome of total HFH and CV death versus placebo (RR 0.75; 95% CI 0.59–0.96; $p = 0.024$).

The prespecified exploratory subgroup analysis of the AFFIRM-AHF[11] displayed that FCM suggestively reduced the primary outcome of total HFH and CV death versus placebo in iron-deficient AHF patients with ischemic HF etiology (RR 0.65; 95% CI 0.47–0.89, $p = 0.007$, for FCM vs. placebo). But, this was not observed in those who presented with nonischemic HF etiology (RR 1.11; 95% CI 0.75–1.66; $p = 0.60$). In contrast to CV death and the remaining secondary outcomes of total CV hospitalizations and CV death, time to CV death, time to first HF hospitalizations or CV death, and days lost due to HF hospitalization and CV death (all p interaction > 0.05), observed a significant subgroup interaction for the secondary outcome of total HFH (p interaction = 0.038).

In contrast to previous studies that found improvement in symptoms, clinical prognosis, and quality of life regardless of HF etiology in CHF,[2,3] this is the first study to identify the interaction between HF etiology and the effect of FCM injection in this AHF population. Only 20% and 17% of the cohort population in the FAIR-HF and CONFIRM-HF trials, respectively, have a nonischemic etiology, making them possibly underpowered to detect an effect in the nonischemic subgroup. The apparent lack of FCM efficacy in the nonischemic fraction may be attributable to the heterogeneous nature of nonischemic HF, which includes valvular and congenital heart disease, which may be the primary prognostic factor, resulting in a reduced sensitivity to detect the effect of intravenous FCM in this subgroup. Second, the lower primary event rate in the nonischemic group (42.8 vs. 78.7 primary endpoint events per 100 patient-years in the placebo arms of each subgroup) decreases the likelihood of observing the treatment benefit with FCM in comparison to placebo.

It is essential to keep in mind that this is a subgroup analysis with limited statistical power and is therefore regarded as hypothesis-generating. The results of this study may have significant public health and financial implications. If validated by future research, guidelines might restrict the indication for FCM from all patients to only those with iron deficiency and ischemic causes of HF. Importantly, this study demonstrates that the administration of intravenous iron during hospitalization for acute HF decompensation is safe and possibly most efficacious in patients with ischemic HF who have a history of HFH. As with important HF medications, there may be a shift toward commencing intravenous iron at discharge rather than delaying until the next follow-up in this subgroup.

ARTICLE 5

Outcome of Heart Failure Management in a Multidisciplinary Clinic: A Randomized Controlled Trial

Pant BP, Satheesh S, Pillai AA, Anantharaj A, Ramamoorthy L, Selvaraj R. Outcome of heart failure management in a multidisciplinary clinic – A randomized controlled trial.
Indian Heart J. 2022;74(4):327-31.

Abstract

The incidence of re-hospitalization in heart failure is a significant problem, and disease management by a multidisciplinary heart failure clinic (MDHFC) has been shown to reduce re-hospitalization, improve quality of life (QOL), and reduce mortality in the Western population. Still, data is missing from the Indian population. The study aimed to assess the feasibility of setting up an MDHFC and its outcomes in an Indian population.

Methodology and result: This was a parallel group, randomized control, single-center study with 40 patients in each group. Patients in the control group attended the routine outpatient cardiology clinic, and the intervention group attended the specialized heart failure clinic from July 2019 to August 2020. At the end of 1 year, the patients in the intervention group attended the clinic more than the control group, with higher usage of angiotensin-converting enzyme inhibitor/ angiotensin II receptor blocker ACEI/ARB, beta-blockers, and mineralocorticoid receptor antagonists (MRAs). There was a significant improvement in ejection fraction (EF) in patients of the intervention arm than in the control arm at the end of one year (Baseline-30 ± 4.8 vs. 31.9 ± 3.9 at 1 year 31.5 ± 5.4 vs. 28.8 ± 4.1, $p < 0.001$). There was no difference in the mortality between the 2 groups, but a 50% reduction in re-hospitalisation at the end of 1 year.

Conclusion: MDHFC demonstrated a significant reduction in heart failure (HF) hospitalizations and improvement in QOL, functional capacity, and drug adherence.

ARTICLE COMMENTARY

Despite the best treatment, heart failure (HF) patients have a bad prognosis. Almost 40% of patients presented with adverse events within 1 year in the form of either rehospitalization or cardiac death. The aim of this study was to assess the impact of the management of HF patients through a multidisciplinary heart failure clinic (MDHFC) on the reduction of mortality, rehospitalization, and improvement of quality of life (QOL) as compared to a routine outpatient cardiology clinic.

This was a randomized single-center study. Block randomization was done. The intervention group underwent follow-up in MDHFC and the control group was followed up in a routine cardiology outpatient clinic. MDHFC consisted of treating cardiologists, trained nurses, social workers, dieticians, and other specialties on demand. At the time of the visit, proper clinical assessment and timely optimization of HF medication were done to achieve the target dosage as per guidelines. Drug adherence was assessed with Morisky Green Levine's (MGL) drug adherence score. Functional capacity was assessed with a 6-minute walk test (6MWT). QOL was assessed by Minnesota Living with Heart Failure Questionnaire (MLHFQ). The total duration of follow-up was 1 year.

The primary endpoint was a composite of death from any cause and hospitalization for HF. Secondary endpoint included death from any cause, hospitalization with HF, cardiovascular death, drug adherence, QOL, and functional capacity. With the intention to treat analysis, the Kaplan–Meier survival curve and log-rank test were used to see any significant difference in outcome between the two groups.

Both groups had similar characteristics at baseline. The average number of visits was higher intervention group (MDHFC) as compared to the routine cardiology clinic. At 1 year, there was no significant difference between the two groups with respect to primary endpoints ($p = 0.19$). But, the survival curve started separating at 5 months showing a trend toward lesser adverse events in the intervention group. HF admissions were lesser in the MDHFC group at 1 year ($p = 0.04$). QOL, drug adherence, and exercise capacity (6MWT) were significantly better in the intervention group. Achievement of target doses of angiotensin-converting enzyme inhibitor (ACEI)/angiotensin-II receptor blocker (ARB), β-blockers, and mineralocorticoid receptor antagonist (MRA) was significantly higher in MDHFC patients. Similarly, New York Heart Association (NYHA) class improvement was significantly higher in the intervention group.

■ INFERENCE

Since there was the systematic implementation of a protocol to achieve maximum target doses, there was a higher rate of adherence to medication and a higher percentage of patients achieved the target dosage as advised in guidelines. This translated into better outcomes in the form of a 50% decrease in HF hospitalization, and more improvement in NYHA class and QOL as compared to the control group. There was a positive trend toward an increment in left ventricular ejection fraction (LVEF) in the intervention group.

Although there were significantly fewer adverse events in the intervention group at the end of 1 year, there was no difference in mortality. Mortality benefits might not be seen due to the short duration of follow-up. Separation of the Kaplan–Meier curve at 5–6 months between two groups may indicate toward the importance of a longer duration of treatment to show any significant benefit in mortality.

Key messages

- Supervised comprehensive approach in MDHFC improves outcomes in HF patients. By decreasing hospitalization, it decreased the financial burden on the health system as well as on individuals.
- Although long-term follow-up may show a decrease in mortality as well given the stronger benefits and frequent crossovers to MDHFC long-term study plan is less likely to be done.
- MDHFC is in need of the hour for HF patients.

ARTICLE 6

Albuminuria as a Marker of Systemic Congestion in Patients with Heart Failure

Boorsma EM, Ter Maaten JM, Damman K, van Essen BJ, Zannad F, van Veldhuisen DJ, et al. Albuminuria as a marker of systemic congestion in patients with heart failure.
Eur Heart J. 2023;44(5):368-80.

Abstract

Aims: In patients with heart failure albuminuria is common and associated with worse outcomes. Still, in heart failure the underlying pathophysiological mechanism of albuminuria is not well understood. In patients with albuminuria with heart failure, the association of clinical characteristics and biomarker profile with both reduced and preserved ejection fractions were evaluated.

Methods and results: In the index cohort of BIOSTAT-CHF (The BIOlogy Study to TAilored Treatment in Chronic Heart Failure) included 2,315 patients were evaluated and in the independent BIOSTAT-CHF validation cohort (1,431 patients) findings were validated. Defined urinary albumin-creatinine ratio (UACR) > 30 mg/gCr and >300 mg/gCr in spot urines as microalbuminuria and macroalbuminuria, respectively. The prevalence of micro- and macroalbuminuria was 35.4% and 10.0%, respectively in the cohort. During admission patients with albuminuria had more severe heart failure, as indicated by inclusion, higher New York Heart Association (NYHA) functional class, more clinical signs and symptoms of congestion, and higher concentrations of biomarkers related to congestion, such as biologically active adrenomedullin, cancer antigen 125, and N-terminal pro-B-type natriuretic peptide (NT-proBNP) (all $p < 0.001$). In both cohorts, the presence of albuminuria was found to be associated with increased risk of mortality and heart failure (re)hospitalization. The strongest independent association with log UACR was found for log NT-proBNP (standardized regression coefficient: 0.438; 95% confidence interval: 0.35–0.53; $p < 0.001$). On performing hierarchical clustering analysis that demonstrated, UACR clusters more with markers of congestion and less with indices of renal function. Similar findings were yielded by the validation cohort.

Conclusion: Albuminuria is consistently associated with clinical, echocardiographic, and circulating biomarkers of congestion in patients with new-onset or worsening heart failure.

ARTICLE COMMENTARY

A significant number of heart failure patients have albuminuria. The aim of this study was to see the association between clinical features and biomarkers with albuminuria in reduced (HFrEF) as well as preserved (HFpEF) heart failure patients.

This was a post hoc study. The patient population in this study was taken from BIOSTAT-CHF heart failure. The BIOSTAT-CHF trial had an index cohort of 2,516 patients and a validation cohort of 1,738 patients. Patients with LVEF < 40%, BNP

> 400 pg/mL, and NT-proBNP > 2,000 pg/mL were included.

A spot urine sample was taken and the urine albumin-creatinine ratio (UACR) was measured. The patients were divided into normoalbuminuric (UACR < 30 mg/gCr), microalbuminuric (UACR > 30 < 300 mg/gCr), and macroalbuminuric (UACR > 300 mg/Cr) respectively. A urine sample of 2,315 patients in the index cohort and 1,431 patients in the validation cohort was available.

Univariate and multivariate regression analysis was performed for the association of log UACR with various biomarkers, e.g., NT-pro-BNP, urinary kidney injury marker (KIM-1), plasma urea, history of diabetes mellitus, systolic blood pressure, and biologically active adrenomedullin (bio-ADM) and cancer antigen 125 (CA-125). All variables with $p < 0.10$ in univariate analysis were included in multivariate analysis. Cox regression analysis was used to investigate the association of UACR with clinical endpoints of mortality and heart failure hospitalization.

Result: The prevalence of macro- and microalbuminuria was 10% and 35.4% in the index cohort respectively. Albuminuric patients were having higher NYHA class, high systolic blood pressures, higher heart rates, and higher plasma concentrations of biomarkers such as NT-proBNP, bio-ADM, and cancer antigen (CA-125) and were more congested clinically. Lesser number of albuminuric patients were taking angiotensin-converting enzyme inhibitor (ACEI)/angiotensin-II receptor blocker (ARB) ($p < 0.001$) and receiving higher doses of loop diuretics ($p < 0.001$) as compared to normoalbuminuric patients.

In the validation cohort, pulmonary pressures and inferior vena cava diameter (>2.1 mm) were higher in albuminuric patients.

The strongest association of albuminuria was found with NT-proBNP followed by KIM-1. And it was seen across all classes of NYHA and both types of heart failure (HFrEF and HFpEF). Similar results were seen in the validation cohort.

Another finding was that there was no interaction between log NT-proBNP and eGFR. So raised NT-proBNP was not due to decreased renal clearance.

Both diabetic patients and nondiabetic patients showed a similar strong association on multivariate regression analysis.

Albuminuria was associated with higher mortality and heart failure hospitalization in both index as well as validation cohort with a p value <0.001 as shown in the Kaplan–Meier curve.

Patients with albuminuria (micro or macro) had increased mortality and heart failure hospitalization as assessed by Kaplan–Meier survival curves in both index and validation cohorts with a significant reduction in survival probability up to 0.5 at the end of 2 years when compared to patients with no albuminuria.

■ INFERENCE

Albuminuria was found to be associated with worse outcomes in patients with heart failure. The extent of albuminuria was more closely related to the severity of congestion rather than intrinsic renal disease. In animal studies of renal vein ligation, albuminuria was seen when pressure exceeds 18 mm Hg and central venous pressure of >18 mm Hg is a common finding in HF. Moreover, after diuretic therapy albuminuria decreased in acutely decompensated heart failure patients. Similarly, in patients of renal vein thrombosis, albuminuria disappears after reversal of occlusion. Congestion may be associated with endothelial dysfunction leading to increased vascular permeability.

One plausible mechanism may be glycocalyx dysfunction which affects podocyte function in glomeruli leading to proteinuria. Excessive renin-angiotensin-aldosterone system (RAAS) activation in heart failure leads to excess angiotensin in circulation which is toxic to podocytes and hence may be responsible for proteinuria.

Key messages

- Albuminuria in heart failure is associated with adverse outcomes in terms of higher mortality and heart failure hospitalization.
- Albuminuria is strongly associated with clinical signs of congestion and biomarkers of congestion irrespective of intrinsic renal function [no interaction with estimated glomerular filtration rate (eGFR)] and irrespective of comorbidities known to cause albuminuria such as diabetes and hypertension.

REFERENCES

1. Puchalski C, Ferrell B, Virani R, Otis-Green S, Baird P, Bull J, et al. Improving the quality of spiritual care as a dimension of palliative care: the report of the Consensus Conference. J Palliat Med. 2009;12(10):885-904.
2. Anker SD, Comin Colet J, Filippatos G, Willenheimer R, Dickstein K, Drexler H, et al.; FAIR-HF Trial Investigators. Ferric carboxymaltose in patients with heart failure and iron deficiency. N Engl J Med. 2009;361:2436-48.
3. Ponikowski P, van Veldhuisen DJ, Comin-Colet J, Ertl G, Komajda M, Mareev V, et al.; CONFIRM-HF Investigators. Beneficial effects of long-term intravenous iron therapy with ferric carboxymaltose in patients with symptomatic heart failure and iron deficiency. Eur Heart J. 2015;36:657-68.
4. van Veldhuisen DJ, Ponikowski P, van der Meer P, Metra M, Bohm M, Doletsky A, et al.; EFFECT-HF Investigators. Effect of ferric carboxymaltose on exercise capacity in patients with chronic heart failure and iron deficiency. Circulation. 2017;136:1374-83.
5. Ankowska EA, Tkaczyszyn M, Suchocki T, Drozd M, von Haehling S, Doehner W, et al. Effects of intravenous iron therapy in iron-deficient patients with systolic heart failure: a meta-analysis of randomized controlled trials. Eur J Heart Fail. 2016;18:786-95.
6. Kalra PR, Cleland JGF, Petrie MC, Thomson EA, Kalra PA, Squire IB, et al.; IRONMAN Study Group. Intravenous ferric derisomaltose in patients with heart failure and iron deficiency in the UK (IRONMAN): an investigator-initiated, prospective, randomised, open-label, blinded-endpoint trial. Lancet. 2022;400(10369):2199-209.
7. Rocha BML, Cunha GJL, Falcao Menezes LF. The burden of iron deficiency in heart failure: therapeutic approach. J Am Coll Cardiol. 2018;71:782-93.
8. Klip IT, Comin-Colet J, Voors AA, Ponikowski P, Enjuanes C, Banasiak W, et al. Iron deficiency in chronic heart failure: an international pooled analysis. Am Heart J. 2013;165:575-82.e3.
9. Jankowska EA, Rozentryt P, Witkowska A, Nowak J, Hartmann O, Ponikowska B, et al. Iron deficiency: an ominous sign in patients with systolic chronic heart failure. Eur Heart J. 2010;31:1872-80.
10. Rangel I, Goncalves A, de Sousa C, Leite S, Campelo M, Martins E, et al. Iron deficiency status irrespective of anemia: a predictor of unfavorable outcome in chronic heart failure patients. Cardiology. 2014;128:320-6.
11. Sama IE, Woolley RJ, Nauta JF, Romaine SPR, Tromp J, ter Maaten JM, et al. A network analysis to identify pathophysiological pathways distinguishing ischaemic from non-ischaemic heart failure. Eur J Heart Fail. 2020;22:821-33.

Index

A

Abortion 113, 114
Acetazolamide 50-52
    addition of 51
    intravenous 51
Acidosis 73
Acute coronary syndrome 49, 69, 75, 77, 96
Acute myocarditis 41
    genetic architecture of 40
Adverse cardiovascular events 65
Adverse fetal events 114
Albuminuria 171-173
Alcohol septal ablation 84, 85
Ambulatory blood pressure monitoring 122
Ambulatory heart failure trial investigators 45
American College of Cardiology 1, 92, 105
American Heart Association 1, 92
Amiodarone 105
Amyloid heart disease 3
Amyloid transthyretin cardiomyopathy 86
Anemia 8-10
Angiotensin-converting enzyme 112
    inhibitors 3, 58, 68-70, 110
    uptitration of 18
Angiotensin-receptor
    blockers 3, 18, 58, 59, 68-70, 110
    neprilysin inhibitor 3, 58, 68, 70
Aortic stenosis 116
    moderate 11
Arrhythmia 92
    life-threatening 92
Arrhythmic secondary endpoint 36
Artery, pulmonary 135
Artificial intelligence 27, 148, 154
Ascites 50, 51
Aspirin studies 102
Atherosclerosis risk 7
Atherosclerotic cardiovascular disease risk 108
Atrial arrhythmias 17, 86
Atrial fibrillation 4, 65, 86, 101, 102, 104, 105, 145
    presence of 87
    treatment of 105
    uncontrolled 65
Atrioventricular blocks 36
Autonomic control 88

B

Baroreflex activation therapy 131, 132
Basal ganglia 88
Beta-blockers 58, 68, 69, 71
Bioprosthetic heart valves 102
Birth weight, low 113
Biventricular pacing 96
Blood
    pressure
        high 8
        systolic 47, 49, 53, 71, 76, 108
    urea nitrogen 155
Body
    mass index 47, 108, 161
    weight 54, 80
Bradyarrhythmia 95
Brain changes, functional 87
B-type natriuretic peptide 135
Bundle branch block 96

C

Cardiac actin-myosin cross-linking 83
Cardiac arrest, sudden 100
Cardiac contractility modulation 129
    therapy 129
Cardiac death, sudden 35, 36, 89, 90, 92, 98, 99
Cardiac implantable electronic device 43, 44
Cardiac involvement, progression of 94
Cardiac magnetic resonance 32, 33, 87
    imaging 21, 26, 28
    abnormal 93
Cardiac myosin, selective allosteric inhibitor of 83
Cardiac output 125, 127
Cardiac phenotyping 28
Cardiac resynchronization therapy 43, 44, 69, 112
Cardiology 154
Cardiomyopathy 35, 43, 44, 84, 100, 111, 145
    arrhythmogenic 35, 41
    associated genes 42
    childhood hypertrophic 89
    hypertrophic 4, 96
    idiopathic dilated 30
    inherited 40, 42, 96
    nonischemic 39, 96, 100
    peripartum 112, 114
    phenotype-only classification of 36
Cardiorenal syndrome 5
Cardiorespiratory fitness 162
Cardiovascular disease 107
    management of 149
Cardiovascular events, strategies of 101
Cardiovascular illness 85
Cardiovascular magnetic resonance 27, 30, 42, 94
Cardiovascular medicine 148
Cardiovascular outcomes 134
Cardioverter-defibrillator reduces mortality risk 100
Case fatality rate 116
Catheter-mounted balloon occlusion and pump system 139
Central venous pressure 121
Chronic obstructive pulmonary disease 17

Complete heart block 20
Comprehensive cardiomyopathy database 37
Conduction system pacing 95
Congestion 73
  systemic 171
Congestive heart failure 16, 105
  guideline-directed medical therapy 3
Continuous physical activity 140, 141
Coronary artery
  disease 4, 7, 30, 31, 84, 137, 148
  fistula 96
Coronary sinus 44
Coronary vein fistula 96
Coronavirus disease 2019 (COVID-19) 21, 22, 43, 65, 83, 165
  pandemic 165
  survivors 21
C-reactive protein, high-sensitivity 9, 129
Creatine kinase elevation 79

D

Dapagliflozin 46-48
  efficacy of 47
Data monitoring 105
Death 54
  cardiovascular 47
  heart failure related 35, 36
Decongestion 54
Deep learning-based virtual native enhancement 27
Diabetes mellitus 4, 80, 108
  higher prevalence of 84
Diastolic dysfunction 26
  assessment of 25
  severity of 25
Diastolic function 27, 80
Dietary approaches to stop hypertension 161
Diffusion tensor tractography images 88
Digital technology 148
Dilated cardiomyopathy 30, 39, 41
  causes of 31
  initiating phenotypic expression of 42
Direct oral anticoagulants 112

Distinct pathophysiological pathways 109
Diuretic therapy, doses of 73
Dofetilide 105
Dominant mutations, presence of 44
Dose-blinded myosin inhibition 82
Drug therapy 46
Dyspnea 72
  severe 83
  short-term symptomatic 72

E

Echocardiographic functional and structural parameters 79
Echocardiography 21, 25, 27
  transthoracic 17, 33, 116
Edema 50, 51
Effective regurgitant orifice area 16, 17
Ejection fraction 47
Electrolyte derangement 73
Electronic health record 66, 151
Electrophysiology 148
Emotional triggers 88
Empagliflozin 53, 79, 80
  effects of 52, 54
Endocarditis, infective 114
Endothelial dysfunction 77
Estimated glomerular filtration rate 47, 71
European Society of Cardiology
  criteria 42
  guidelines 9
Exercise
  induced ventricular ectopy 91
  test abnormalities 89
  training 2
Extracorporeal membrane oxygenation 119

F

Fascicle, posterior 95
Fatty-acid binding protein-4 110
Ferric carboxymaltose therapy 168
Fisher's exact test 31
Focused cardiac ultrasound 115, 116
Furosemide 55

G

Genetic
  cardiomyopathies 35
  testing 40
Genotype-based classification 35
Global longitudinal strain 23
  score 20
  prognostic value of 22
Glomerular filtration rate 124
  baseline 73
Guideline-directed medical therapy 3, 5, 17, 24, 57, 66, 68, 128, 130, 132-134, 150, 158, 166
  implementation of 58
  management, uptitration of 24
  maximum tolerated doses of 83

H

Heart
  defect, congenital 108
  transplantation 14
Heart disease 74
  ischemic 28
  structural 96
  valvular 148
Heart failure 3, 6, 10-12, 16, 17, 19, 22, 33, 46, 47, 51, 57, 61, 63, 72, 74, 77, 92, 95, 104, 107-110, 112, 113, 124, 127, 134, 135, 138, 148, 153, 154, 156, 160, 162-164, 169, 171, 173
  acute 52, 68, 73, 167
    decompensated 7, 139
    systolic 157
  chronic 1, 8, 46, 49, 61, 165
  composite of 11
  congestive 16, 105
  decompensated 7, 48-50
  diagnosis of 115
  estimated prevalence of 119
  event 54
  exercise capacity for 76
  genetics in 35
  interventions in 134
  management 4, 55, 105, 118
  outcome of 169
  new-onset 24
  nutritional management of 161
  prevention of 6

risk of 4, 6, 107
stable chronic 7
substantial 160
subtypes 111
symptomatic 79
therapy 66, 149
Heart Failure Society of America
    Guidelines 105
Heart Rhythm Society 92, 93
Heart failure with preserved
    ejection fraction 1, 6, 25, 26,
    107, 121, 122, 125, 126, 129,
    161
    treatment of 130
Heart failure with reduced
    ejection fraction 9, 16, 70, 77,
    96, 98, 107, 108, 112, 128, 131,
    132, 150, 158, 161
    treatment of 130
Hemodialysis 65
Hemodynamic trial 125
Heterogeneity 35
Higher vasopressor 14
High-grade atrioventricular block
    21
High-intensity interval training 2
Hydrochlorothiazide 48
Hyperkalemia 70, 71
Hypertension 84
    arterial 122
    chronic pulmonary 74
    pulmonary 74-77, 113, 125, 155
    severe pulmonary 114
    treatment 108
Hypertensive disorders 109, 116

I

Idiopathic cardiomyopathy,
    assignment of 30
Implantable cardioverter-
    defibrillators 90, 92, 94, 98,
    100
    guidelines for 92
    implantation 36
        selective criterion for 44
Implantation failure 95
Implanted left ventricular assist
    device 56
Indian Heart Rhythm Society 102
Infertility 107
Infiltrative disorders 4
Inflammatory condition 41
Inotropic agents 49

Interdisciplinary Network Heart
    Failure 157
International Normalized Ratio
    87, 102
International Society of
    Thrombosis and Hemostasis
    102
Interventricular septum 121
Intrauterine fetal demise 114
Intravenous ferric carboxymaltose
    164, 165, 167
Invasive testing 3
Iron deficiency 9, 10, 164, 167
    prognostic significance of 8
Ischemic cardiomyopathy,
    assignment of 30
Ischemic left ventricular
    dysfunction 136, 137
Ivabradine 112

K

Kansas City Cardiomyopathy
    Questionnaire 130, 135, 144,
    145, 155
Kaplan–Meier survival curve 170
Kidney
    disease, chronic 17, 73, 145
    injury marker 172

L

Late gadolinium enhancement
    25, 27, 28, 31
    detection of 28
Left atrial
    diameter, measurement of 17
    function 16
    volume 33
    index 25, 59, 130, 142
Left bundle
    branch
        area pacing 96
        block 36, 45
    fascicle pacing 95
Left ventricle
    ejection fraction 11
    end-systolic dimension 80
Left ventricular 20, 23, 87, 128
    assist device 118, 152, 163
    implantation 35, 120, 121
    support 152
    use of 36
    dilation 30

dysfunction 143
ejection fraction 3, 11, 46, 47,
    52, 61, 67, 69, 77, 80, 83,
    93, 94, 107, 109, 110, 121,
    130, 135, 137, 150, 151, 155,
    165, 170
    estimation of 26
end-diastolic
    diameter 45
    pressure 123
    volume 80
filling pressure 32
    catheter-based assessment
        of 33
global longitudinal strain 21
outflow tract 82, 83, 85
septal pacing 95
systolic
    dysfunction 39
    function 44
Left-dominant arrhythmogenic
    cardiomyopathy 35
Lipoprotein, low-density 110
Liver
    disease, chronic 145
    failure, end-stage 65
Loop diuretic therapy 51
Low-density lipoprotein 110
Low-sodium diet 65

M

Machine learning 148, 149, 152,
    154
    applications of 154
Major adverse cardiac events 13,
    129
Major ventricular arrhythmia
    35, 36
Malignancy 4, 17
Malnutrition 161
Maternal cardiac events 114
Matrix metalloproteinase-3 110
Mavacamten 84
    therapy 83, 84
Mean ejection fraction 65
Mean oral furosemide dose 49
Mean serum potassium 71
Mechanical circulatory support,
    use of 13
Median estimated glomerular
    filtration rate 49
Median N-terminal pro-B-type
    natriuretic peptide 49

Medical therapy 19
Mesenchymal precursor cells 127, 128
Mineralocorticoid receptor antagonist 68, 70
Minnesota Living with Heart Failure Questionnaire 133, 170
Mirabegron 76
  treatment 76
Mitochondrial dysfunction 8
Mitral regurgitation 116, 134, 135, 142
  functional 16
  quantified 16
  secondary 146, 147
Mitral valve
  prolapse 114
  transcatheter edge-to-edge repair 146
Multicentric longitudinal study 86
Multidisciplinary heart failure clinic 169
Multiple sclerosis 116
  severe 114
Myocardial dysfunction, subclinical 21
Myocardial infarction 27, 102, 129
  acute 12, 13, 79, 88
  recurrence rate of 14
Myocardial recovery, machine learning-based prediction of 152
Myocardial scar 27, 30
  quantification of 28
Myocardial tissue, immunohistopathology of 42
Myocardial tuberculosis 96
Myocarditis
  acute 41
  prevalence of 43

N

National Health Service 42
Natriuretic peptide 3
  elevation 59, 60
Nephrotic syndrome 73
Neurogenic bladder dysfunction 75
New York Heart Association 45, 82, 97, 114, 130, 132, 135, 142, 155, 156, 170

Nitrates 53
Nonheart failure-related hospitalizations 135
Noninvasive techniques 33
Nonspecific intraventricular conduction delay 95, 96
N-terminal pro-brain natriuretic peptide 123, 126
Nutrition assessment 160
Nutrition disorders, high prevalence of 160, 162

O

Obesity 161
  central 4
  paradox 161
Obstructive coronary artery disease 149
Obstructive hypertrophic cardiomyopathy 82-84
Omecamtiv mecarbil, effect of 61
Oxygen saturation 76

P

Pacemaker 21
  implantation 85
Peak atrial longitudinal strain 16, 17
Pearson Chi-square 31
Percutaneous coronary intervention 17, 136, 137
Permanent atrial fibrillation 78
Phenotypic heterogeneity 35
Phosphodiesterase inhibition 77
  ameliorates endothelial dysfunction 77
Pleural effusion 50, 51
Polyunsaturated fatty acid 162
Post-left ventricular assist device 120
Post-myocardial infarction period 80
Postrenal sympathetic denervation 123
Potassium levels 50
Preeclampsia 4
Pregnancy
  medical termination of 114
  outcomes 113
Pre-heart failure 59, 61
Prerenal sympathetic denervation 124

Preserved ejection fraction 1, 48, 79
Programmed electrical stimulation 93
Prosthetic heart valves 17, 113
Pulmonary arterial wedge pressure 126
Pulmonary artery 135
  pressure 156
  systolic pressure 78
Pulmonary capillary wedge pressure 121, 123
Pulmonary hypertension 74-77, 113, 125, 155
  different subtypes of 155
Pulmonary vascular resistance 126, 127
Pulmonary vein isolation 105

Q

Quality of life 54, 85, 104, 105

R

Randomized controlled trials 131, 153
Rankin scale score, modified 118
Reduced ejection fraction 11, 75
Refractory angina 17
Remote hemodynamic-guided heart failure management, effects of 155
Renal compression 124
Renal disease, end-stage 56, 65
Renal dysfunction 124
Renal failure, acute 54
Renal impairment 84
Renal sympathetic denervation 121-123
Renal tamponade 124
  hypothesis 124
Renin-angiotensin-aldosterone system 150, 173
  inhibitor 151
Rheumatic heart disease 101, 102, 114, 116
Rheumatic mitral stenosis, moderate-to-severe 102
Rhythm control 105
  ablation-based 104
Right heart
  catheterization 33, 78
  failure 120

Right ventricular 20
  dysfunction 24
Rivaroxaban 101, 102

S

Sacubitril, effect of 59
Sarcoidosis, cardiac 92, 94, 96
Self-directed exercise training 2
Sensitivity analyses 43
Septal fascicle 95
Septal myectomy 84, 85
  merits of 85
Septal reduction procedures 85
Septal reduction therapy 82
  referred for 83
Septal scar 96
Serum ferritin 9
Serum iron 9
Serum potassium 71
Serum sodium 65
Several organic anions, presence of 73
Severe acute respiratory syndrome-related coronavirus 2 21, 22
Sex-specific risk factors 4
Shock, cardiogenic 12, 13, 49
Sildenafil 78
  effects of 76
Single premature ventricular contractions 90
Singular phenotype platform 35
Sinus rhythm 105
Six-minute hall walk distance 77, 130, 132, 133
Six-minute walk test 170
Sleep disorders 4
Society for Cardiovascular Angiography and Interventions 13
Sodium, dietary restriction of 63
Sodium-glucose cotransporter-2 48, 79
  inhibitor 4, 46, 112, 151, 166
Sotalol 105
Speckle track echocardiography 17
Spironolactone 70
Standard guideline-directed therapy 75
Stillbirth 113
Strain echocardiography 20
Stress leads, context of 88
Stroke, composite of 102
Structural heart disease 96
  evidence of 47
Structural tractography connections 88
Structured exercise training 2
Sudden cardiac death 35, 36, 89, 90, 92, 98, 99
  incidence of 92
  prevention of 93
  primary prevention of 98
Superior vena cava 139
  intermittent occlusion of 138
Surgery, cardiac 85
Swan–Ganz catheter 155
Systemic embolism 86, 102
  prevalence of 86
  risk of 86
Systemic vascular resistance 126

T

Takotsubo syndrome 87-89
Temporary mechanical circulatory support devices 14
Thalamus-amygdala-insula 88
Thromboembolic phenomenon 86
Thyroid, uncontrolled 65
Tolvaptan 72, 73
  right space for 73
Torsemide 55
  loop diuretic strategy of 56
Transcatheter edge-to-edge mitral valve repair 142, 143
  renal sympathetic denervation 123f
  repair 134, 147
Transcatheter mitral valve replacement 146, 147
Transcatheter tricuspid valve intervention 140
Transendocardial mesenchymal precursor cell therapy 127
Transferrin 9
  saturation 9
Transthyretin amyloid cardiomyopathy 86
Tricuspid
  annular plane systolic excursion 24
  regurgitation 25, 116, 140, 144
    severe 141, 145
  stenosis 116
  transcatheter edge-to-edge repair 144, 145
  valve
    intervention techniques 141
    surgeries 145
T-test 31
Two-dimensional speckle-tracking software 23

U

Uric acid 73
Urine albumin-creatinine ratio 172
Urogenital infections, active 80

V

Valsartan 59
  effect of 59
Valve
  disease, primary 17
  replacement 85
Vasoconstriction 77
Vasodilators 53
Vena cava, superior 139
Vena contracta 17
Ventricular assist device 14
Ventricular ejection fraction 44
Ventricular pacing, increased frequency of 45
Ventricular tachycardia 94
Virtual care team group 58
Virtual native enhancement 28
  technology 29
Vitamin K antagonists 87, 102
Volume overload, clinical signs of 50, 51
Volumetric cardiac magnetic resonance imaging 59

W

Weight loss 54
Wild-type transthyretin cardiac amyloidosis 86
Women's Health Initiative 108
Worsening heart failure, combined risk of 47